Lose weight eating the food you love

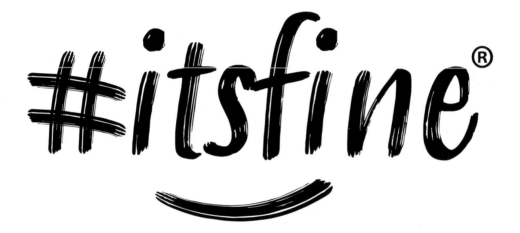

#itsfine®

BEN SMITH AND PETER ANDRE

SEVEN DIALS

First published in Great Britain in 2023 by Seven Dials,
an imprint of The Orion Publishing Group Ltd
Carmelite House, 50 Victoria Embankment
London EC4Y 0DZ

An Hachette UK Company

1 3 5 7 9 10 8 6 4 2

A CIP catalogue record for this book is
available from the British Library.

ISBN (Hardback) 978 1 3996 1011 7
ISBN (eBook) 978 1 3996 1012 4
ISBN (Audio) 978 1 3996 1694 2

Printed in Italy

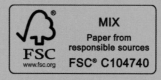

www.orionbooks.co.uk

contents

Introduction

ABOUT US

peter andre . . . entering the world of nutrition

Many people will know me, probably from the TV, or perhaps from that song . . . you know the one. But what everyone doesn't know is how badly I have suffered with my mental health around food. Not just as a result of sustaining my famous six-pack, but also from trying to lose weight by following some of the worst fad diets out there.

From a young age, I was obsessed with many goals, including the achievement of a perfect 'ripped' physique. But at what cost? Despite physically looking the picture of health, I was often run down and unwell due to the combination of my long and hectic work schedule and lean, low body-fat physique. I was obsessed with every single food I put in my mouth. A diet with almost zero fat, eating the same meals day in, day out: broccoli, chicken and rice. Not only did I miss out on a host of vitamins and minerals, but I didn't account for the physical effects of combining my diet choices and pursuit of perfection while burning the candle at both ends. Once dubbed 'the hardest working man in pop', I would work, work, work, but not fuel myself properly to be able to sustain that. And, when I did eat, it was so low in calories that I would often feel fatigued, using only adrenaline to keep myself going. A lot of you who have achieved your weight loss goals through following a fad diet can probably relate to this.

My appearance was always a feature in the media and it came with a huge amount of pressure to maintain it, essentially doing whatever it took. It's actually a pressure many of us feel today in modern society, don't we? But, as you can imagine, very much amplified when in the public eye.

No matter how determined we are, we can't keep doing things in such a restricted way as it will always end up taking its toll. For many years, I felt I had nailed it regarding what I would eat, when I would eat it, how much I would train, etc., with all my spare time focused on work. But eventually I rebelled against the very thing that I had strived to achieve. Like many of us, I became a yo-yo dieter, with substantial splurges of binge eating followed by periods of low calories, zero carbs and tons of exercise. I became great at sticking to this plan and would almost tailor my 'good' or 'clean' periods of eating around key photo shoots, to give the impression of myself in perfect physical and mental health. But it couldn't have been further from the truth.

So, in my thirties and fed up with this cycle, I just went for it, going on a binge that didn't just last days or weeks but, in fact, lasted for over half a decade. The more I was pictured during this time, the more my emotions and negative relationship with food drove me to eat. However, I still maintained that outward happy persona, just styling myself with larger clothes, hoping to make the weight gain less obvious.

As I continued through my thirties, I looked for a weight loss solution, but in all the wrong places. Initially I tried to revert to old ways with a bland, bodybuilder type way of eating, to get back to being as lean as possible. This didn't work, as the cravings would get the better of me within a few days, so would be followed by huge episodes of self-sabotage. The overriding urgency of rapid fat loss consumed my mind and I tried several well-known fad diets out of desperation which, at best, I stuck to for six months. All the while I was yo-yoing up and down on the scales, developing an obsession with the number shown and using that to determine my success. The reality was, despite achieving short-term weight loss success, at the end of each year I either weighed the same or even more, and the impact of this on my mental health was significant.

I was in such a mess! Trying anything and everything I could to lose the weight and missing out on so much life with friends and family. All because of my obsession with weight loss, which, in the long run, led to me getting nowhere. I knew there had to be a better way and, as I came closer to my forties, I went looking for it.

For me, the shift in mindset initially started by changing my goal. Health became the number one priority. Not how good I could look walking along the beach but how good I could feel instead.

This was a huge turning point for me, because it allowed me to move away from the scales and focus on what was important. It removed the urgency to lose weight that I had focused on for so long.

I was then able to look at my lifestyle, how I lived day to day, and made sure that whatever I did from that point onwards was not just enjoyable but sustainable, which, of course, was the complete opposite of how I'd behaved around food up to that point.

What became obvious quickly was that each day could be very different, in terms of free time, location and the facilities/foods that were available to me. No wonder I struggled to eat in line with a rigid and strict eating plan, because my lifestyle could never accommodate it, which is often the case for so many people.

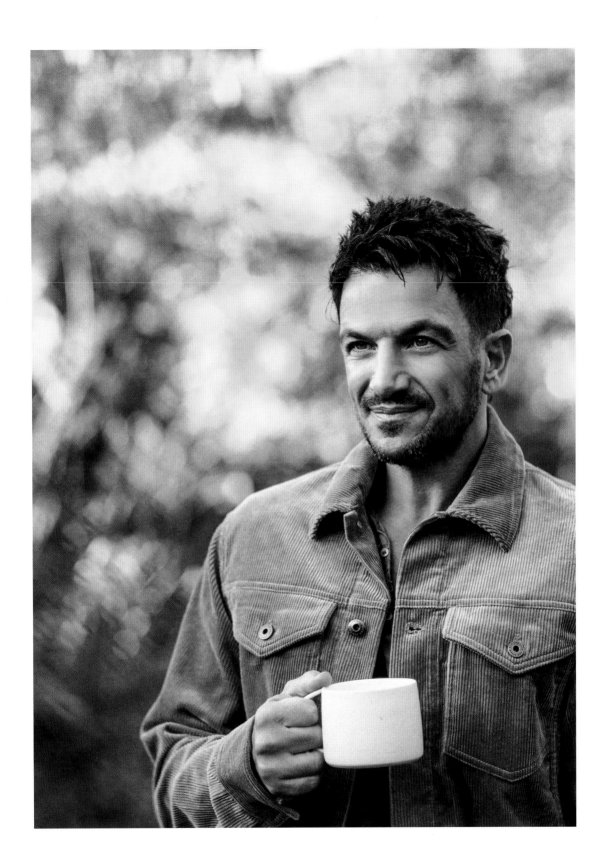

I decided to take a flexible and balanced approach to achieving my goals, making a seven-day period my target rather than a 24-hour period. Some days I skipped breakfast, some days I didn't eat much until mid-afternoon. Some days I ate three meals, some days I snacked all day until having a larger dinner, but throughout the process I stayed accountable and kept track of my calories for each week.

To get into the swing of things took a few months. Those old habits and feelings of guilt would kick in, but I remained focused and true to the process as I knew it was perfect for me. Months went by and I not only started looking and feeling great physically, but also mentally. All by saying 'it's fine' to what I wanted!

I faced plenty of obstacles along the way, which in the past would have almost certainly resulted in me throwing in the towel due to going 'off plan'. Instead, I overcame them. Not with some magical low-calorie meal or way of eating, not at all. It was just by getting back to a normal balanced way of eating, making a choice not to weigh in to assess the 'damage', but instead reflecting on how nice the meal was, the time spent with family and friends and how far I had come.

Through my forties, I went through a life-changing experience, successfully maintaining what I see as the best shape of my life. By shape, I mean the complete package of health, fitness and true food freedom with a positive relationship with food.

Of course, #itsfine® didn't exist then, only in my head. The way I monitored, tracked and maintained what I did week in, week out, was done manually. There was nothing out there that facilitated the weekly balanced approach I had used. That was, of course, until I came across Ben online, who had just released a beta (test) version of an app and concept I was very passionate about.

After using the app for several months I honestly believed he was on to something big, so I put together an email in the hope we could have a chat about his plans. From our first conversation I was hooked, not just because I loved the app, but because Ben's passion to help people was so infectious. Once he explained to me how big of a problem he was trying to fix, I knew I wanted to be part of getting this information out there and felt I had a new purpose in my life within the world of nutrition.

so who is ben smith then?

From a very early age, I was known for two things – my fascination with bodybuilding and nutrition, and my appetite (my parents even called me the 'human dustbin'). In other words, I loved food and lots of it!

Throughout school, I was very much into the gym. Despite eating a large amount of food, I always seemed to look fit and healthy. Outwardly yes, not quite with the abs of Pete, but in great shape and full of confidence. But, behind closed doors, that couldn't have been further from the truth. The problem was, in the 1990s, young men didn't sit down and share anything other than talking about the girl they'd kissed at the cinema or which nightclub they should go to that weekend. Come to think of it, even today, issues around food and mental health still aren't discussed enough.

I was in a constant battle against a huge appetite and being a fan of a nice takeaway, but desperately wanting to obtain the lean, bodybuilder physique of my dreams. In my mind, that couldn't be achieved without a restrictive diet of chicken, rice, broccoli and sweet potato, so everything I enjoyed was firmly off the menu. I began to see food as function and not taste, with protein intake being the number one priority. I was obsessively weighing each ingredient to make sure it wasn't even 0.1 of a gram above or below what I wanted.

Despite all this, my body never really changed. Why? Because what people didn't see was the frequent relapses behind closed doors. Mainly during the evenings and weekends, where the lack of variety, flavour and satisfaction got too much for me and I'd have enormous binge eating sessions, consuming up to 15,000 calories at a time. All that hard work just couldn't be sustained, and it always resulted in mammoth blowouts at the weekend. It was then back to a further five days of complete restriction, back on the chicken and rice, with double workouts, but getting to Friday weighing and looking the same as the week before. Zero physical progress and yet infinite amounts of mental damage.

Throughout my twenties this pattern continued, sometimes I was having much longer binge eating episodes and gaining a few extra stone, and then covering it up by telling everyone I was 'bulking' and there was nothing unusual here. It was all just part of my 'plan'.

The irony was that I had also been working during that entire decade as a personal trainer and nutritional therapist after qualifying in my late teens, helping clients to achieve amazing results. However, not seeing similar results myself just caused the depression to build and build. *Was there something wrong with me?* I thought. With that I started to reduce the carbs almost completely, eat even more protein and remove anything remotely 'bad' from my diet. Until, that is, I had the biggest binge of my life that wouldn't last just a weekend, but for most of my late twenties and early thirties.

There was no trauma behind it, no event that set it all off. In fact, I'd met the love of my life and started a fantastic new job that still allowed me to work with my nutrition clients via Skype. But my personal relationship with food had taken me to such a dark place that I just rebelled against it all, giving up my quest to obtain a 'perfect' physique and instead eating anything and everything I wanted.

I was a huge takeaway fan and, having seen them for so many years as being counterproductive, wrong or naughty, or having used them as a 'cheat meal', I just went into self-destruct mode after every one I ate. Slowly but surely, I found I was eating takeaways every single day!

Being 5'10" tall and now weighing in at over 300lbs (over 21 stone), I was classed as morbidly obese. I was at the point where I couldn't do the simplest of daily tasks, like going to the loo properly, walking up stairs, showering or putting on socks. I was struggling and had lost all my confidence in my own journey, but all the while was very successfully working with my nutrition clients remotely.

Despite several attempts over a few years to lose the weight, and now in my thirties, I struggled to get into any form of momentum and structure. The same pattern of rapid weight loss (28-42lbs/2-3 stone) was always followed by even faster weight gain, taking me back over the 300lbs mark.

With the birth of my son Alfie, who unfortunately needed regular stays in hospital every couple of months, and my wife becoming disabled, with a host of rare and misunderstood conditions, food was becoming more and more of a comfort blanket and a way of dealing with stress. I decided that I needed to free up my time and move into a new job working from home, which would enable me to be there much more for them.

As 2012 came around, I needed an operation to repair a nerve issue in my wrist, which I thought would be very straightforward. The actual procedure was straightforward, but the hospital was reluctant to do it until my very high blood pressure was back within normal range. So, I crash-dieted and, within six weeks, got my weight down enough to be able to have the op. The day of the operation, after kissing goodbye to Cara and Alfie, I made a promise to them that I would be a better husband and father and get all the weight off. Lying in hospital, I looked back on all the times my weight had stopped me doing so many things with Cara and Alfie. At this point, I felt unstoppable in my head and knew that a few months after my op I'd be in that gym, strictly following a calorie-controlled regime 24/7 and would be in the shape of my life!

All healed and after setting up a makeshift gym in my garage, I was ready to get going. I created a complex spreadsheet detailing all my calories for the day, as well as my macronutrient ratios showing protein, carb and fat consumption targets. I set myself a goal of losing 140lbs (10 stone) by the summer of 2013.

During this intense period, I became a recluse, barely leaving the house other than for the school run. Every day was the same. Getting up at 6 a.m. to do an hour on the treadmill before work, then meals prepped, job, back in the home gym for weight training and then repeating the same process. Alfie was in hospital half a dozen times during this period, as well as Cara, but I kept true to sticking 'on plan'.

During the spring of 2013 I achieved my goal and, aside from loose skin around my stomach, I was happy with my physique and felt confident in how I looked. Having come from such a dark, lonely and unhealthy place with my body, I initially felt happy and, with that, had an even stronger desire to help people reach their weight loss goals. So, with the support of Cara, I began working for myself full-time as a nutritional therapist.

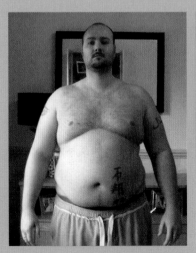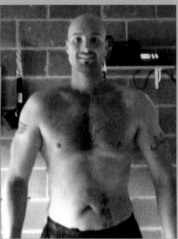

Despite creating plans that were helping hundreds of people, I began struggling again myself. At first, I blamed it on the long hours but, deep down, I knew the real reason. When I looked back to the moment I stepped on those scales and saw that magic number, just a few days after this I had the stark realisation of what my life was going to look like to maintain those results. Instead of feeling proud and positive about moving forwards, I felt scared, worried and anxious about eating out, going on holiday and trying to hit my daily calories and macros all the time.

I spent most of 2013 following a slightly relaxed version of what I'd been doing, introducing a 'cheat meal' every Saturday, which worked for a few months, but it slowly crept into a 'cheat weekend'. Despite personally struggling, my client base grew and grew, taking me to the point where I had to turn new enquiries away. Frustrated with this, I went back to my software roots, using technology as a way of removing some of the admin involved in delivering tailored plans and the need to see me in person for support and advice. Within a few weeks, I realised that I could create a slick, personalised process that would go on to genuinely help hundreds of thousands of people all over the world reach their health and fitness goals as well as support them through their journey.

Clocking up long working days and spending many hours answering thousands of emails, I had zero time to live the obsessive lifestyle that got me to lose the weight in the first place. Not only that, I was now suffering from a depression that came in the form of imposter syndrome, where I didn't feel worthy enough to be in a position coaching people through weight loss. But my empathy and experiences of being morbidly obese just kept me going, and this sense of purpose drove me to work harder and harder over the next few years as I was so emotionally attached to the process of helping people.

The negative impacts of my seriously deteriorating health alongside my obsessions with food and my business had made life very difficult for me. I was not only suffering myself but was causing suffering to those around me. At that point, I knew I had to leave my passion behind to focus on getting better.

September 2017 was a very important date in my mind because Cara and I had planned to get married. Tipping the scales at the heaviest I'd ever been and with serious mobility issues, the thought of limping down the aisle in a custom-made XXXXL suit petrified me. However, a lack of confidence with how I looked was the least of my worries because, after waking up in the middle of the night gasping for air, I went to the doctor for a full check-up, which revealed a list as long as your arm of health concerns. I was on the cusp of Type 2 diabetes, I had serious gout and the onset of sleep apnoea. Not only that, I also required a hip replacement and the reattachment of an elbow tendon. I was in a mess! I felt lost, alone and frightened at this point and knew I had to sort this out once and for all.

I had to be honest with myself in order to look into an area that most men in particular didn't dare delve . . . mental health. After seeing various psychologists and specialists in this field, the diagnosis was clear. My negative relationship with food had given me a condition known as 'binge eating disorder'.

All I had ever done was focus on how fast I could shift the weight. I didn't care how I achieved it, just that I would do whatever it took to get there in a specific time frame. I realised that I had to move away from this mindset and change the goal from weight to health, replacing the obsession of a target date with a long-term goal of sustainability. I needed to be able to find a solution that would be achievable, not just for the short term, but forever.

Calories had always been an important part of what I believed in. After all, there is no question that fat loss comes from eating less energy than your body needs. But did it have to be so obsessive, did it need to be so frequent? This theory made me look at other parts of my life and how it could complement areas that I had previously ignored or categorised as bad or negative. I started to embrace things I liked doing, such as having a takeaway, or the fact that some days I just didn't fancy breakfast, making sure that flexibility was at the forefront of how I designed my plan moving forwards. Ultimately, I took the approach that I would say 'it's fine' to anything I wanted to eat, in line with a calorie target range that I would aim to reach by Sunday evening.

Could this be the answer for me? Could doing the complete opposite of what I did before really help my mental health and finally leave binge eating behind for good? It was worth a shot. When it came to meals, I focused on nutrient density, enjoying plenty of carbs, fats, snack items and the flexibility to change my mind at any time. I wanted to take my arch enemy of a takeaway and turn that into an anchor that kept me grounded each week, but also not see it as a reward or a cheat. I believed that the key to moving away from guilt and self-sabotage was to make sure I regularly included the so-called 'treat' foods, but then also ensured the day that followed was just a normal day. Being normal around food, like my friends and family were, was at the top of my list of goals and I believed I could get there by following this plan.

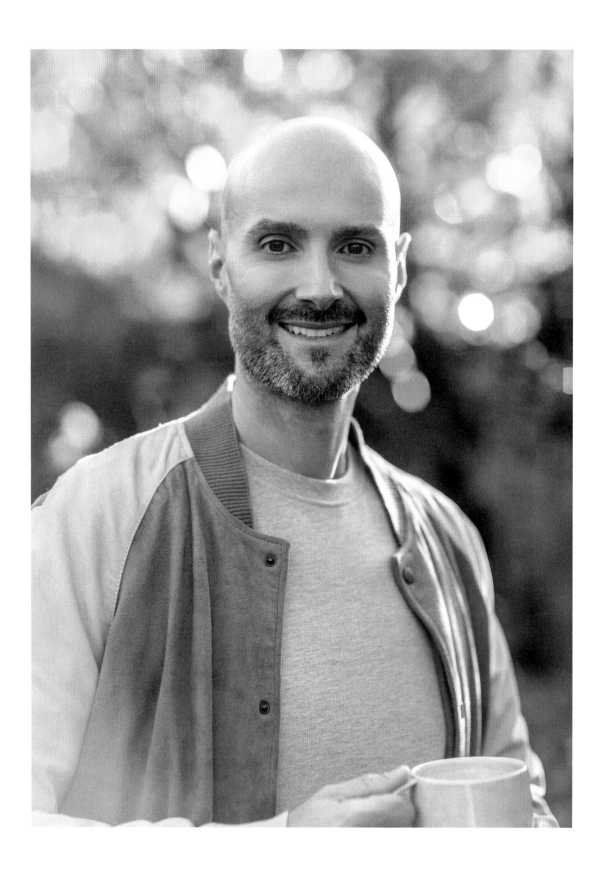

The first few days were awful. My natural instinct was to start doing exercise straight away, but my fitness was terrible and I was so riddled with injury that I really struggled. I started walking on the treadmill and using the recumbent bike but, after just 10 minutes, I felt excruciating pain in my hip and lower back and had to stop. This was my first obstacle to overcome, so I took the approach to create a weekly target that didn't include any exercise at all. This meant a little less food but, with that, less pressure on me, which was a real positive. Any exercise I did do just meant MORE food if I wanted it.

The adjustment to eating something that had been so 'off plan' and forbidden meant I had loads of mind games to face. Each one was a fresh new battle to contend with, but each time I got past it I grew mentally stronger, week on week. Not using the scales as a form of progress validation was so refreshing. Instead, I only stepped on them once a month with my eyes closed, using the camera to capture the number, refusing to look myself. Of course, I knew I was losing weight, but my sole focus became how I felt mentally. Celebrating the little wins each day with the food I ate and the way I behaved made me feel so content.

Not a week went by where I hadn't enjoyed a takeaway with my family or a meal out with friends. No day was ever the same set of meals or the same set of circumstances either. Life was unpredictable and it was OK because I was not accountable day by day. And, no matter what happened, I said 'it's fine'.

Within a few months, little things started to feel like habits, almost subconscious. More so than anything, I noticed a change in how I felt just before and just after making impulsive choices. Not worrying about what I was going to eat, just going with it, and then after, not even thinking about it. These moments were breakthroughs for me and were building a new foundation for my ever-changing mental health.

Being no stranger to weight loss, I got to a point close to my wedding where I felt it was time to go for the final suit fitting. It was at that point, when I fitted perfectly into 32-inch trousers (when previously 52-inch were too tight), I decided to weigh in on the scales and take a look, finding myself right back to my ideal weight, over 140lbs (10 stone) lighter. Although pleasing, that moment created very little sense of achievement for me as I felt I was merely at the start of my journey. Now the hardest part was about to begin – maintaining the results.

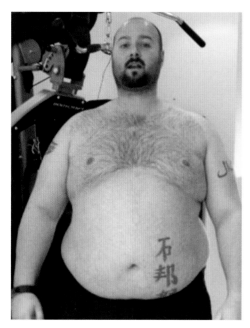 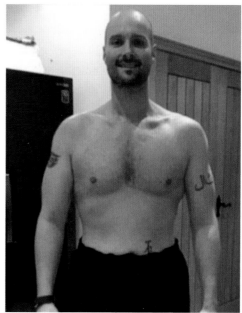

Months went by and I continued with my new, flexible approach to food and was now at the longest period for decades of being binge-free. Friends, family and old colleagues kept encouraging me to share my new approach to weight loss with the world, but I kept saying that until I had lived this life and maintained it for eighteen months, I wasn't going to advocate the approach. I wanted to be 100 per cent sure.

In 2018 and following a conversation with my best friend, John, who I had employed as my right-hand man previously to run customer support, we decided to return to the health and fitness industry. Our aim this time though was not just to help people lose weight but to rescue them once and for all. John didn't need much convincing; he loved the industry and had seen how incredible my approach was. Together we began working on bringing the ethos to life and started what would be a three-year journey of creating #itsfine.

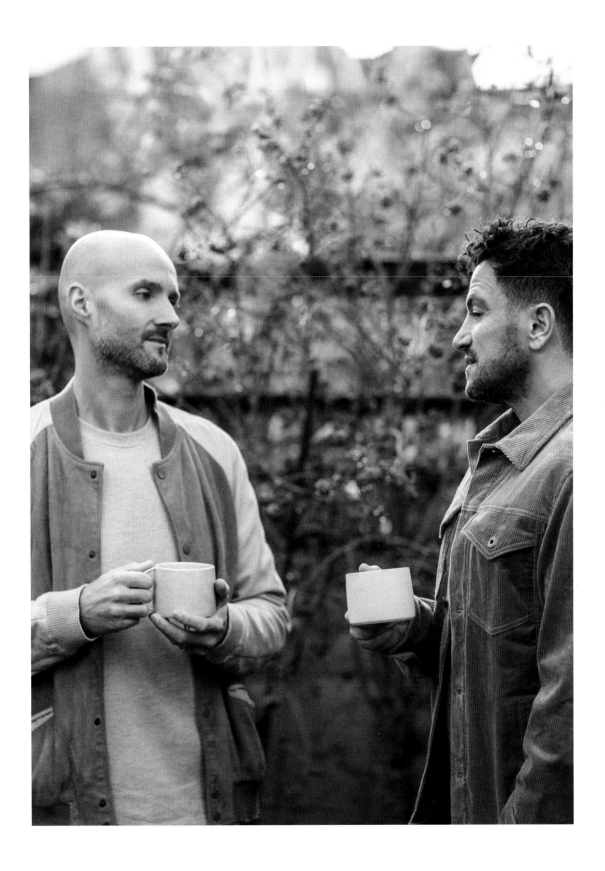

Chapter 1

IF DIETS DON'T WORK, WHAT WILL?!

so how do I lose weight then?!

It's a question we hear all the time. And no doubt you have been searching for the answer for years. The funny thing is, the answer was right in front of you all along, you just needed someone to show it to you.

The root cause of the issue is fad diet culture! So, to answer the question, you need to understand that everything you've been taught by diets NOT to do, the things they told you were incorrect, that would negatively affect your weight loss journey and take you 'off plan' – well, they were wrong.

So, from this point onwards we want you to say two words to all of these myths. And they aren't 'I can't' or 'It's wrong'! But instead, with a big smile on your face and with complete confidence, say #itsfine.

We want you to say #itsfine, because the main reason for not being able to achieve your weight loss goals is because of self-sabotage, which is caused by those negative thoughts that creep up in your mind about you and your ability to lose weight. Those negative thoughts fed to you by the nonsense that is fad diet culture.

You're told you ate something 'off plan', which in turn undermines your efforts and progress, so you give up. It's not because you haven't got your calories right, it's not because you're not exercising enough, it's not because you have a slow metabolism and it's not because it's your fault.

You have been conditioned to believe that food is either good or bad, right or wrong, and this sets you up for failure from the start. Food should be happiness and enjoyment, as well as both a planned and spontaneous choice.

Based on our experience working with so many people, we can confidently say that we know you. We really, really know you. Because we have been you.

We know that you have spent years yo-yoing up and down with your weight on the scales.

We know that you just want to feel and behave 'normally' around food instead of over-analysing everything that goes into your mouth.

We know that you want to feel happiness around food instead of guilt, worry and anxiety.

And we know you need rescuing, and that's what saying #itsfine will ensure happens.

how will this work?

So, what if we told you that you can eat anything you like and lose weight?

Well, you'd probably not believe us, would you? And if you did believe us, you would ask HOW?

Of course, the how is the really important part, because this is not achieved from reading one sentence and magically losing 7lbs (½ stone) in a week. It's achieved by going on your own journey of discovering who you are and what you enjoy, because the only plan that will work for you, the plan that we want to help you find, is unique to you. Once you discover that, you can move forwards feeling positive and confident.

Now don't get us wrong, your weight loss journey will be challenging, but it will also be something you never thought possible . . . enjoyable!

The first step is always to take your dieting beliefs and wipe the slate clean for a full reset. But we appreciate that's a tough nut to crack, so we will take it step by step, using a method developed over years of working with thousands of people just like you.

Each chapter of this book will focus on a popular dieting myth and will show you why it is, and always has been, false. These are the small steps designed to help you towards building a new foundation for a strong, long-lasting result. Later in this book, you will find delicious recipes containing many of the things you've been told are off limits, as well as being packed full of nutrient-dense ingredients.

That is the key, to focus not just on physical health through nutritious food, but also on mental health by giving you the confidence to enjoy all foods and not be scared or anxious about them. By using this positive mindset approach, you will have all the tools you need to move forwards.

This is why we created #itsfine, to be both an empowering message of food freedom and also an insight into nutrition which, when combined, forms our unique formula for sustainable weight loss. Because in order to be rescued from fad diets, it isn't as simple as saying 'eat less and move more'. That's actually one of the most negative things you can say to someone who has a bad relationship with food. Portion control is vital to ensure the body burns fat, but we wanted to simplify the concept of daily calorie counting and make it much easier to follow.

what to expect

We want to manage expectations from the start because, in an industry full of smoke and mirrors, we pride ourselves on honesty and transparency. It's the unrealistic expectations that diets have sold you in the past that contribute massively to why you quit and fall off the wagon time and time again.

Think about it. One day you're eating anything you want and completely overindulging. Pizza, sweets, crisps, burgers, you name it. Then the next day, you're expected to not only cut all those things out, but to starve yourself. Because, supposedly, that's how you lose weight.

For some reason, you have to accept this as being the only way to 'diet' and 'lose weight', even though your common sense knows there's a lack of any kind of strategy and no sustainability for long-term results.

Let's look at fitness, for example. You decide that you want to get fitter, but you don't start by running a marathon, do you? You go for a walk for 15 minutes for a few days, then a gentle jog for 10 minutes for a week, then achieve a run for 30 minutes, and that continues. In other words, you gradually build up to getting fitter. And, eventually, a marathon would be a realistic goal. A challenge, yes, but a more realistic one.

Can you see how crazy diet culture is then and how it promotes these unrealistic expectations? You expect, with no practice whatsoever, to change years of negative eating habits literally overnight, then keep this up forever. When you find that it's not working and you hate it, you try to convince yourself to keep doing it out of desperation for the 'promised' quick results. You trade off what you see as short-term discomfort because you believe it will result in long-term gain. Sound familiar? Sound like something you might repeat again and again?

But what if there was a different way, a way that didn't mean you had to go through those types of struggles?

With that in mind, we'd like to tell you what to expect with this book and we think it's going to surprise you, as it's a bold statement. **You can expect to achieve your weight loss goals faster than ever before!**

You're probably thinking 'Well, how much will I lose then and in what time frame, because this sounds amazing?!' So, let's put some substance behind that statement and give you some perspective on what we mean.

Ask yourself this question: 'Have you ever lost a large amount of weight in one week?' I bet the answer is yes. Then ask yourself: 'Have you put most of that weight back on again, perhaps 90 per cent of it?' The answer again is probably yes. That process gets repeated constantly over the course of a year and all you end up losing overall is, in fact, a few pounds. But you don't focus on that, do you? You focus on those moments you see as a success, where you lost half a stone in a week. You cling on to that process and feeling of accomplishment as your ongoing strategy to achieve your long-term weight loss goal.

With all that in mind, if we were to try and sell you something with a sales pitch along the lines of 'lose 14lbs (1 stone) in 6 months', you probably wouldn't consider it. Even though the reality is losing the weight at a steady pace over half a year, with slight but consistent drops on the scales each month, is infinitely faster than a year of rapid losses and gains, which leave you no closer to your end goal.

So, although it seems like we're asking you to accept the process as being slower than you want, what we're really asking you to do is honestly look back on your previous weight loss journeys and realise that we are now going to take you through the fastest weight loss of your life and ensure you stay there, forever.

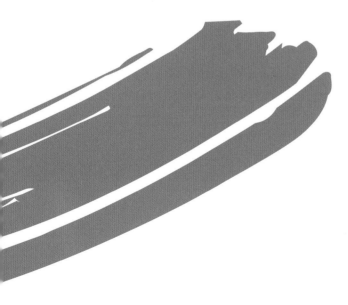

an introduction to portion control

OK, you will know what we mean by portion control and it's not that you don't understand it, it's the fact that you either don't want to use it or you don't stick to it long enough to see that it works. Sticking to the process and being consistent with it was the biggest problem we wanted to solve.

You need to shift your perception of what food means for your journey. The type of food you eat is not important for fat loss to occur, but it's vital to ensure that you're able to stick to your plan and make sure, once you achieve your goals, that you're able to sustain them. We always say, if you're doing something now that you can't see yourself doing in a year's time, then you're doing it wrong.

One of the biggest challenges we face in the world of nutrition is trying to re-educate. It's so much easier to teach from scratch, as re-education means that you first need to understand and accept what you have done in the past hasn't worked. Only then can you move forward knowing what you need to do next to be successful – but is this true?

You're probably already aware that if you eat less food (energy) than your body needs, your body will have no choice but to find that energy elsewhere – from stored body fat. This is the only way you will ever lose body fat and no magic pill, formula or food type will work in place of this, only in conjunction with it. So why do you ignore that fundamental piece of factual information, do the opposite and remain a consumer of fad diets?

Our aim, therefore, is to re-introduce you to portion control, but with an approach that is easy to follow and is combined with the goal of achieving food freedom.

what is food freedom?

Have you ever heard the term before, or even believed it's achievable? Well, it's the definition of what saying #itsfine to the food you want to eat will achieve, by removing all the strict everyday rules that control your life in big and small ways.

Food freedom gives you your life back. It stops you from obsessing day to day about what you have eaten, didn't eat, or want to eat but 'can't'. When you say #itsfine, it becomes life-changing and opens up a whole new world to you. You suddenly have the ability to fully engage in your relationships, with social events, moments of spontaneity, your hobbies, your life!

To be able to, with complete confidence, say #itsfine to anything you want to eat along your weight loss journey is the ultimate goal. It does take time and effort to shift the mindset to this way of thinking, but it's the lack of emphasis on building a positive relationship with food that has been key to you failing to sustain your results. It's totally overshadowed by quick fix, instant diets that don't address the root cause of what got you to where you are. Leaving you constantly taking one step forward and two steps back.

Consider this example. If you were bad with money but you didn't have much of it, imagine what you'd be like if you had loads of it. You'd just go on a spending spree, wouldn't you? If you have a bad relationship with food now when you can't afford to, imagine if we gave you a magic pill to lose all the weight instantly. What do you think would happen now you're at your goal weight? It wouldn't be long before you ate something that you weren't supposed to, which leads you to feeling guilty and spiralling out of control and regaining all the weight.

The very first step on this journey is to understand that all food is equal and it's not to be viewed as good or bad. And remember, you're not on your own on this journey. We are here with you, and you're already taking that step right now.

This is so important for you right now. In fact, it's THE most important thing, but it can't be rushed into. You can't expect to wake up one day with a whole new perspective on food and be able to intuitively eat anything and everything, feeling happy and confident. That would be great, but that's an advanced position to be in that takes years of building good habits to achieve. What you need is to just make a start, and actually taking the first steps can be the hardest part of the journey. But when the plan is clear and so much more enjoyable, you will feel a lot more comfortable to get going and that's where we come in.

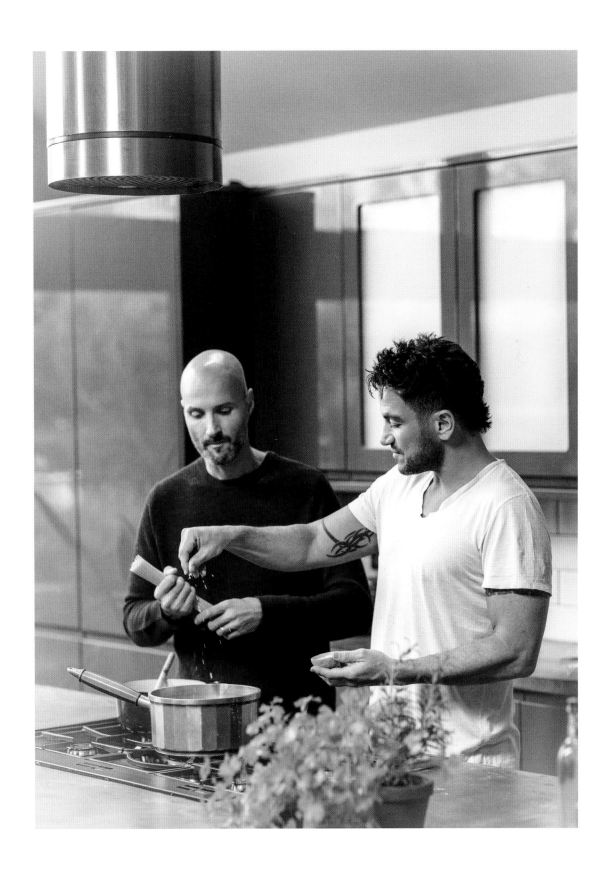

Chapter 2

HOW DID I GET HERE?

asking the right question

This chapter is about addressing the elephant in the room. Rest assured, although this chapter is taking you on a journey of self-discovery, it's nothing heavy and it doesn't require hours of deep thought. We already know the answer, so trust us when we say it will be a real eye-opener and will give you the facts you need to move forward.

So how many times have you sat down and thought to yourself 'How did I get here?'

No doubt you all have, and no doubt you will have spent years, decades even, pondering the when, what and how of your predicament.

We have asked this question ourselves thousands of times over many years, to thousands of people! And in almost every circumstance the initial answers are similar, and the actual answers are almost always wrong. But why?

It's because a lot of people don't see the complexity behind the question, and if you don't understand the question, you'll never find the right answers or start addressing the real problem so you can move forward.

So don't think of the question as 'How did I put on so much weight?' – this isn't what you need to answer. Not looking how you want or weighing what you want is just a by-product caused by something much greater that isn't because of your upbringing or childhood, for example, but something you learnt much later on in life, in adulthood. Of course, when we are feeling down or stressed we often respond to that with food, but we also do the same thing in moments when feeling the complete opposite and on top of the world.

Carrying excess body fat will have a negative impact on physical health, but that can be caused by a lack of activity, a different career path, or even something as simple as returning from holiday and feeling a little uncomfortable. In these moments, very simple progressive changes could have been applied and soon you'd have been feeling much better about yourself. However, you didn't do that and instead went down a different route altogether.

So, let's rephrase it . . . 'How did I develop a negative relationship with food?'

What we want you to think about is not when you first felt you had a problem with weight, but when you realised you had a negative relationship with food. Which, by the way, you still may not even realise you have.

Let's dig deeper into the question. At what point in time did your eating become disordered (restrictive, compulsive, irregular or inflexible)? When you stopped being mindful about fruit, vegetables and general health and started analysing every single ingredient you ate? Or, when you started consuming foods you didn't like specifically to lose weight, as recommended by someone else? What about when you ate something and felt bad about it because someone told you that you should? Don't forget, of course, those times you woke up panicking, trying to come up with a strategy to counteract what you ate the day before.

When did all this happen? It's nearly always down to a fad diet . . .

You can probably still remember it, right? An email, a leaflet, participating in a group session, a referral from a colleague, or clicking a button on the internet. That impressive promise combined with a motivational picture. 'Lose the weight in XX days' or 'Burn fat and get in the shape of your life'. It was at that moment that you began your journey down the wrong path, yet it seemed so perfect at the time. The reality is, for most of you, it will have sneaked up and caught you off guard, often when you were at your weakest or most vulnerable and susceptible to the promise of a quick fix.

Most of us are reluctant to admit to ourselves that we were wrong. Sometimes that's just what you need to do though and facing it head-on is key here. You are just one of many millions of people all over the world that had no or limited experience of nutrition and wanted fast and easy improvements. Who wouldn't go for that, right?

It's not nice to realise that what claimed to be the answer to your problems, actually created them in the first place, and for so many of you, it has had a hugely negative, ongoing impact on your quality of life.

Looking back on what triggered that new thought process and conditioned you mentally to think negatively about food is important. When you know what it was, then you can feel confident that you're addressing the root cause. A moment of realisation that everything done in the past following fad diets has not only NOT worked, but has actually made the situation worse.

So saying #itsfine is as much about eating and doing what you enjoy as it's about taking your life back and knowing that, from this point on, everything will be OK. You are at the start of a fresh new journey now, where the approach is not only evidence-based, but transparent. Your expectations will be managed properly from here on in and we will guide you carefully throughout.

when did it all start?

Having realised now what created the problem, let's focus on why you chose to go down the dieting route. How it felt at the start, and when that first day was. Let's get you remembering what you initially experienced and unwrap how what seemed like such a positive step towards achieving your goals only took you further away from them.

Whether it was a moment on a beach, walking past a mirror, being in the gym or just reading a magazine, something caused you to think so negatively about your appearance that you felt it necessary to seek help.

To make matters worse, you probably stepped on to a set of scales to see a number that was higher than you expected or greater than a Google search suggested was normal for someone your gender, age and height, for example.

We get it! Everyone is critical of themselves and wants to be better in some way physically. At this point in the game, you could have made some simple lifestyle choices, remained consistent with them over time and made improvements over the course of a year. However, we live in a world of fad diet culture where that approach is just not acceptable. Well, it certainly feels that way, doesn't it? It seems so slow, it takes time and effort, and we want results yesterday, so don't even consider a sensible plan of action. We reach for the products that claim they'll get you there quickly with seemingly no effort at all.

So that's day one, but, and we can't stress this enough, at this point in your journey you really didn't have a significant issue with food. It's likely you were just the friend with the larger appetite, or the one with the desk job that didn't like the gym, or you just felt a little squidgy that day and happened to open a magazine to see a chiselled fitness model's ripped six-pack or a slim, toned model on holiday.

Now try to imagine a world without fad diets for a second. If you were in that world, feeling as you did in that first moment, what would you have done? Would it have looked like any of these?

1. *Overall, just reduced the amount of food on your plate perhaps*

2. *Cycled or walked to work*

3. *Started consuming more fruit and veg*

4. *Joined a tennis club*

5. *Joined a gym*

6. *Skipped a meal or a snack*

Perhaps some of you would have done one of the above, others a few of them. They aren't right or wrong, they are just options. Depending on you, your lifestyle, your likes and dislikes, your job, etc., they would either be an ideal fit, or they would be difficult to achieve, but the decision would have been yours, no one else's. No outside influence, no flashy sales pitch, just common sense and things most people would have thought of and added to their own list. The important thing to remember here is you'd have looked at your own life and made sure the options suited it.

But we don't live in that world, sadly. So common sense, reflecting on your own personal circumstances and free will just go out the window, because you see a faster route to success. Plus it comes with a photo of that same chiselled model on holiday to prove it! They didn't do anything on your list, they just ate a special combination of foods that supposedly ramped up their metabolism and got them fit, slim and toned in a few weeks.

At this point, for you, being more active and moving a little more each day would have been a great starting point. Combining that with being more mindful about reducing processed foods, eating more fruit and vegetables and getting enough protein would have helped you significantly. You would have felt better and no doubt would have started to see that you looked better. You're probably thinking, wow, how simple does that sound, and at that moment it would have been. However, that advice was never given to you because it's not that same money-maker, it's not shown in the places we normally look. If we do find it, we try it for a very short period of time and get impatient, then before you know it, there's a new model on the scene who appears in the following month's edition of *Slimmer You* magazine and you want to know more.

It's made worse by that same social media-driven fantasy we all fall for. People are quick to shout about their successes, but often remain silent about their failures, and this couldn't be more true in the world of fad diets.

The big, popular, commercial weight loss brands have such a significant reach that in almost all workplaces, groups of friends and families, you'll find someone who is currently being successful (in line with the product's own guidelines) or who has restarted and is feeling good about themselves. So not only have they attracted your interest with a strategic campaign, but you have a friend to do it with, or a friend of a friend of a friend who looks amazing now – all within a seemingly short period of time.

So, you decide to give it a go. You fill out the form, they've told you that you're wobblier than you should be and set you a nice generic weight target. At this point in your life two huge changes occur, massive changes, in fact, that will shape your life forever.

1. *Food now has a function other than health and enjoyment, and it's broken down into two categories: GOOD and BAD.*

2. *That number on the scales is everything to you. It's not about how you look and feel, but it's all about that number and, without fail, it MUST always go down!*

You didn't have these rules in your life before, ever. But now they are there, and if you deviate from them, you fail. Wow, how aggressive is that at the start of something new and daunting?

Have we exaggerated? If you have been incorporated into those fads, then you will know we haven't. But as you reflect, the funny thing is that those same people who introduced you to them never once mentioned that in their testimonial? However, you've paid your fee and you've committed, so you move forward with the plan.

Can you remember the lead-up to your first day on that new regime? Can you remember what you did? Well, we bet we can and we weren't even there!

The trouble with how diets label food as 'good' or 'bad' is that pretty much all 'bad' foods taste nice! And in a lot of cases, they taste much better than 'good' foods. So, faced with a period where you can't eat things you really enjoy the taste of, what do you do the day before? You binge! You have an almighty blowout, so anything goes and you eat until you feel fit to burst. A process we refer to as Last Supper Syndrome. Another lovely gift we can thank fad diet culture for. The scary thing is, for most people, this is the first time they will have ever experienced a negative relationship with food, and sadly, that relationship grows from strength to strength from there on in. Not only have you been told verbally that food is 'good' or 'bad', but you've also just felt it through eating it, with not half as much enjoyment as you thought. So, you had the initial panic combined with excitement, followed by enjoyment, then, towards the end, feeling, well, a bit rubbish. No wonder, as you've just eaten a week's worth of food in a day.

Diets love you to do this, and for two reasons. The first being weight, more specifically your starting weight. Your results are determined from the get-go by a reduction on the scales, so they want you to be as heavy as possible. Most people start fad diets on a Monday (you'll have been there), because it's neat and because it leaves the weekend wide open to overindulge before the big day. In most cases, the foods you will have consumed will be made up of lots of sugar and salt and eaten right up to bedtime. Not only have you got an awful lot of undigested food in your stomach, but you will be retaining a lot of excess water due to your body using it to store unused energy (carbohydrates).

The second reason is that you'll be feeling rubbish after the 'bad' food and, therefore, you're more likely to be focused on eating the so-called 'good' stuff, despite the fact that it might not suit your taste buds. It feels healthier and better for you, what's that word they throw around . . . cleaner . . .

Your day one arrives and you weigh in at around half a stone heavier, so you're now even more determined to lose weight. Week one goes OK. The food, albeit not much of it, was restrictive, from packets and fairly processed, with odd combinations as part of the 'on plan' guidelines, but was just about manageable. You get to the end of your week and hop on the scales to discover you've lost over half a stone! WTF! That's amazing. Do you remember this?

But from this point on, things start to get very stressful and progress starts to change almost randomly. You have now put a huge amount of pressure

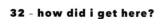

on yourself to repeat the same results again, or certainly close to it. Weight loss = success, after all, so all you need to do in order to keep making progress is just what you did the week before. Pretty soon you're going to hit your target of a 28-lb (2-stone) loss! Just stick to the plan and the funny foods and you'll get there, right?

How did it go from there? Was the second week a fraction of the first week's loss? Did you second-guess everything and then move into daily weighing to see if your new food tweaks, as suggested by the fad diet guidelines, worked any better? Did some days go up on the scales, despite you eating the same thing the day before when it went down? It's not a pleasant journey and it doesn't leave you feeling great.

Sadly, the most common knock-on effect at this confusing stage is a blowout! You blame yourself, because the diet obviously works, just look at those success stories that you keep getting shown. So, it must be your fault then, because the first week was amazing. Never in your life had a feeling of failure resulted in an episode of binge eating and you have now done it twice in a month – at the start of something that was meant to help you achieve your goals, and now again after just four weeks.

Can you remember what you felt like after that second blowout and what you did next? If it's anything like the many people we have met, you went back to the one thing that caused the problem in the first place and restarted it. In your mind, you held on to that first week believing it can happen again, and sure enough it did, but that is a cycle of highs and lows, ups and downs, binges and restarts, which has been the norm for you now for years and you have never managed to escape its clutches . . .

We just want to pause here, because it sounds like a telling-off! But it really isn't meant to be that. Remember, we have done this, too, and been sucked in. This type of mindset is taught and we all learnt it. But what can be learnt, can be unlearnt, which is the starting point of what we do to get you saying #itsfine.

we know who you are, but do you?

We only exist because of a desire to help people just like you. And not just over the short term, because the journey you need to go on takes time, effort and consistency. Funny that, all the things that fad diet culture tells you isn't needed. You wouldn't have found us had you not embarked on a fad diet in the first place, but you did and you're now ready to start the processes of trust, resetting your mind and true self-discovery around food and health.

Not only have we worked with thousands of people like you, but we were you! That's why we care, because our goal is to disrupt the fad dieting industry for the better, and take people through our, up until now, unheard-of method. You see, you may feel like you're in the minority, a fad diet failure among a sea of success stories, but let us just assure you that you are, in fact, in the majority. It's very rare to find anyone with a truly positive relationship towards food and their body, so please don't think you're broken compared to the rest of us, you aren't.

So, who are you? Well, first of all, you are brave. Brave because we are the polar opposite of everything you have ever done, all that you have experienced and learnt. So even contemplating our approach is something that pushes you massively out of your comfort zone.

From here on in you need to be honest about what you really want and need. Draw a line under what you have been led to believe will happen with weight loss, because with #itsfine it won't. Don't get us wrong, the end result you're aiming for will, but just not in the same way as you've come to expect. We focus on truly tailored nutrition and helping you to build a plan that suits your life perfectly, taking the time to get it right, so that you can then move forward enjoying the process with fresh new goals in mind.

Goals are very specific and personal to each person, but we would like to set the first three for you. At first this can seem a little unusual, but you will soon realise that you'll want to achieve them more than anything, because we know you. We have detailed a little table for you to list yours alongside our first three and remember, these are both short-term and long-term goals. People can lose sight of what's important along the way, especially if they have a 'moment' when things just get a little too bumpy in life. This is completely normal, of course, and is part of every weight loss journey, so we'd like these three goals to serve as a reminder of the bigger picture and what you really want out of life.

1. <u>To feel normal,</u> which, in our opinion, is the biggest goal. To just be and feel normal around food. To eat something without a care in the world, no judgement, no worry, no over-analysing. A lot of you will have friends who seem to always look the same and just eat food and get on with each day. They may have a meal out with you and never once talk about dieting or weight, and take it for what it is, a fun, sociable time. They don't do anything different the next day and they don't feel any different, as they have a much healthier relationship with food. This is very much the end game with what we do with you. But it's important to keep this in mind and to recognise moments when you do this, as they are huge wins and often go unnoticed when you get in the swing of things.

2. <u>Being impulsive</u> . . . We are going to teach you that recipes are just a guideline and, although ours have reasons behind the ingredients we have used, changing, removing and swapping things is part of what you need to do to get comfortable around making food. It will also ensure that your taste buds are fully satisfied, your budget is considered, and allergies and intolerances are easily managed without worry. We also want you to feel confident when asked out for a coffee and muffin, offered a piece of cake in the office or wake up one day and just fancy something else. Because in all those circumstances you will see #itsfine. When you understand that it's not the combination or type of foods that will get you to your goals, you will start to feel a sense of food freedom. In the world of fat loss, no food is magic, so we want to expose all the lies you've been told by fad diets you've followed in the past.

3. <u>Weighing in</u> . . . a lot less! Before you go taking a hammer to the bathroom scales, hold on a second. It's not the scales that are the issue, it's just the way you have been told to use them. How you allow them to dictate your mood for the entire day based upon your body's relationship to gravity. Deep down, if you really think about it, frequent weigh-ins are annoying, stressful and pointless, adding no value to your life at all. Without a doubt, when done correctly it can serve as one of the many markers of progress, but we need to get you away from daily and weekly weigh-ins. We totally understand that this will be tough. Let's face it, it's a deeply ingrained habit that's going to be hard to break, but it's so important you do. We'll talk about this more during Chapter Six, so this is just a mental warm-up for now. But trust us when we say relief and empowerment are the most commonly used words from our members once they start measuring progress in the ways we suggest.

List everything down there, what the goal is, when you went to achieve it and why, no matter how big or small it can seem, or how irrelevant to dieting it may seem. Put a new focus on achievements that are as far away from scale weight as possible. These are called Non-scale Victories, or NSVs, and ensure you feel a sense of accomplishment week in, week out. Trust us, the knock-on effect that having a positive relationship with food can have on all areas of your life is unbelievable, so go all out! When you say #itsfine, anything is possible. From curing Type 2 diabetes, feeling more comfortable through the menopause, finding the confidence to meet someone or getting a promotion at work. Finding happiness with food and living day to day with freedom of choice alongside structure and consistency will change the way you feel about yourself and the positivity you put out there.

your goals

WHAT	WHEN	WHY

take your life back

We will have covered some things already that you may have found a little overwhelming, a bit intense perhaps, but it's all about bringing the truth about your relationship with food to the surface and showing you the real problem and cause of it.

Now you are ready to press on with #itsfine and focus on the future. The past is the past and there is no looking back for you now as you start this new journey with us. It's exciting!

Chapter 3

SELF-SABOTAGE

so, what does self-sabotage mean to you?

Notice that we aren't asking you if you have experienced it, as we can say with absolute certainty that you have. Simply because it's the number one reason why people fail on fad diets . . . Just ponder this question for a moment – apart from any diet you've ever done, can you think of a time when you have quit something for absolutely no real reason?

Let's give you an example of what quitting for no real reason may look like. Let's say you're driving in a car with your route set out to your planned destination. However, halfway through the journey there is an obstacle, a road has been closed, which means you need to follow a diversion instead. Rather than just taking a different route, using some unexpected changes that will still get you to where you're looking to go, you decide to slam on the brakes, do a U-turn and go back to the beginning. You've never done that in your life, yet on your fad diet plan you do it constantly.

In this scenario, what would be even worse is if you decided you were going to follow the diversion but your passenger friend convinced you that, as you've come off the planned route, you might as well just not bother, go back home and start fresh tomorrow. You then ignore your instincts and common sense, and do as they suggest.

You can think of the planned route in this example as your fad diet. It can get you to your destination, but if life crops up and throws in something you weren't expecting and you have to change your plans, you're suddenly doing something wrong. Add into the equation the person sitting next to you, who could be a representative of that diet, or a friend who has also been sucked into that one perfect route but has been back to the start many times. They see that slightly different way as scary, as something you just can't do and still be successful, so they convince you not to take it.

But ultimately what you need to remember is that you would still get to your destination, no matter what route you took. Some diversions can last for a minute or so, and others go on for miles, but you're still heading in the right direction.

What we are trying to emphasise here is that going 'off plan', any plan in life for that matter, happens only as a result of an inflexible and badly designed plan. A plan that is unable to take into account you, your needs, your likes and dislikes, and more importantly, your lifestyle.

There is a very simple starting point that you need to embrace and accept, which is that everything is on plan. So that everything that could happen to you, good or bad, planned or random, is part of your life and is part of your plan to achieve your goals.

Earlier we asked you to identify the reason and the moment that your negative relationship with food began. We did that to ensure you could move forward with perspective and an understanding of your situation. Well, we now want you to make a promise to yourself, and to us, and we're going the whole hog with it and asking you to sign for it. No pencils please, we want this in pen, because there is no going back now. It's time to commit to saying #itsfine and the way we do things long term.

I, _____, promise from this point on to commit to a

complete diet reset and dismiss and forget everything

I have previously been taught to believe is the best way to lose

weight. I appreciate this will be tough at first, but I will

be open-minded and trust in #itsfine and never

use the words 'OFF PLAN' again.

Signed:

_____

Have you signed it or are you having a cheeky read on? If not, get squiggling, because being fully committed is a must and is what it takes to fix years, maybe even decades, of conforming to fad diet culture.

Well done! You've committed now, but don't be worried. Yes, it's normal to feel a little apprehensive about starting even small new things, and this is a big one. But you will remember this moment in months and years to come and be thankful you did.

When you break down the true definition of self-sabotage, it's quite intense and seems very drastic. That's because it is, yet it's formed the norm within the fad dieting world and is totally accepted and brushed under the carpet!

Self-sabotage on a fad diet happens when you dismantle yourself deliberately, mentally and emotionally, resulting in you hindering your own success by undermining your long-term personal goals and values.

In its simplest form . . . you jack it all in because of a piece of chocolate, ignore any past successes and quit for no reason . . .

It really is no reason and we want you to list below all the times you can remember self-sabotaging and why. We want all the undeniably ridiculous experiences you have had to be there in black and white, right in front of you. We've heard them all, so don't be shy, none of them are wrong. So much so that we are going to list the top three most crazy reasons we have come across.

1. I was poorly and bought some cough sweets. I felt terrible as I'd had some sugar and being on a no-carb diet had shut down the fat-burning process anyway, so I just bought a load of sweets until I felt better.

2. I just found out my kitchen scales were faulty which means the meals I've prepped won't be accurate. I've ordered some more and will restart then.

3. I forgot to track the calories today, so I'll start fresh tomorrow.

We could have listed hundreds of them and actually you may be about to put similar ones on your list. Now it's your turn:

REASON	OUTCOME

So, take a moment now to read all your reasons for self-sabotage. Some of them will stand out as being a bit daft and you can't believe what made you throw in the towel. But others, still to this day, you would consider doing again and almost see them as being a valid reason for quitting. We see this all the time and know that it's due to being told that what you have done is bad, but with no justification. There is no reason given as to why it was wrong, you're just told that it was, so you believe this and feel all you can do is quit.

What happens is that self-sabotage, when repeated over and over again, becomes habit and habits are tough to break. To break this cycle and build new habits, you've got to BELIEVE. Believe that a) the reasons you self-sabotaged were wrong and unjustified, and b) saying #itsfine to all those reasons will actually get you closer to your goals.

You see, this is why we asked you to put pen to paper and commit. We are asking you to do something very challenging, especially when you have invested so much of your life, time and money into fad diets for so long. It can feel almost like your religion is being questioned and you can get quite defensive about that at first – we experience this all the time. However, the only way you can break free is to understand that everything you have previously been told was right is, in fact, wrong.

It's now time for us to expose and explore the reasons behind self-sabotage so that you can feel comfortable about saying #itsfine when they happen.

how do you lose body fat?

Do you know the answer to this? What we find interesting is that pretty much everyone does, or at least has some idea that involves the concept of portion control. That's not what you eat though, it's the amount of food that goes on a plate and gets eaten that will determine how you look. Therefore, if there's not a lot on the plate, the chances are you'll lose weight. If it's piled high, you will gain it. Would you say that's an accurate description?

What's funny is that every single fad diet you have ever done has either chosen to ignore that or even told you it's inaccurate, and you have believed them. We know this, because, having a fundamental understanding of portion control would have prevented 95 per cent of the reasons why you quit.

When you're desperately trying to lose weight, you're often mentally at your weakest and susceptible to things that throw common sense out of the window. Fad diets know this. Let's put it like this. Fad diets have actually convinced you that 1+1 does not equal 2 in the world of food, and that's something we are going to need to correct so that you can build upon an accurate foundation of understanding. It's time to dip into the world of calories . . . and they aren't confusing at all.

We use calories very differently to everyone else, which will be explained later on in the book. For now, it's important to lose the negative stigma around calories, because understanding them is what will enable you to feel comfortable saying #itsfine and give you the validation that whatever caused you to give up before was nonsense.

Before we press on with this, there is something important to mention, but at this stage in the game isn't too relevant. Some of you will have heard of **nutrient-dense foods** before and others won't, but here is a brief overview of what that means.

nutrient-dense foods

Think of nutrient density as getting the best 'bang for your buck'. In other words, the most nutrition from your calories. Nutrient-dense foods contain vitamins, minerals, complex carbohydrates, healthy fats and protein. Examples of nutrient-dense foods include fruits and vegetables, wholegrains, full-fat dairy products, wild-caught seafood, grass-fed meats, eggs from pasture-fed chickens, legumes and nuts. Processed foods, on the other hand, tend to have much less nutrient density to their calories. Calories from alcohol have even less and are known as empty calories. In other words, you can have foods that still give your body the same measurement of energy but without much goodness.

If you never gave the above much thought, you would still lose body fat. You wouldn't feel great, but you would lose body fat. The plan that we put in place for you and the recipes we provide you with as part of a balanced approach take care of all that stuff for you. We are not looking to turn you into nutritionists, but we do want you to understand the basics that fad diets never focus on.

Now calories, very simply put, are a measurement of the energy contained in food. We needed a way of measuring this to ensure our bodies were getting the amount of energy needed to survive. They were not invented as part of a diet plan. In fact, they were first used back in the nineteenth century when weight loss would have been the last thing on people's minds. They should not be seen as good or bad, they are just a name for a measurement of energy and a tool that can be used.

If you consume more energy (calories) than your body needs it will have no alternative but to store the excess. This is what happens when you eat what is called a calorie surplus. Bear in mind excess calories from ANY food will be stored as fat in the body. But if you consume less energy (calories) than your body needs, eventually it will use your body fat to meet that energy requirement. Meaning, and this bit is extremely important, **being in a calorie deficit eating any type of food will result in your body using its fat stores as energy**. It's worth noting as well that if you meet your body's energy demands perfectly (maintenance calories) you will maintain your current weight, regardless of what food you eat.

When it comes to food, your understanding of what is right or wrong needs to change and this is where calories are useful. This is because, in the past, eating something forbidden, 'off plan', wrong, ignited the urge to self-sabotage. There really is no such thing and calories prove this for you. So purely from a mathematical perspective, is there any difference at all between a bowl of porridge amounting to 500 calories or a bacon sandwich amounting to 500 calories? Stop over-complicating things and thinking about the macronutrients and nutrient density for a second, just think about the numbers . . . For you and your journey, the answer is no. You're not a biochemist doing research on how the body digests and processes energy from different compounds. You aren't an Olympic athlete wanting to optimise performance through nutrition. You're somebody who needs a little insight and some perspective into portion control to help you move away from diet culture.

Half of what we are telling you is what you already knew way before you started any fad diet and probably still know, deep down. You have just lost sight of it. We get that, but we don't shy away from it. We just make it easier to understand and apply.

If a person chooses to create a recipe being mindful of calories, or creates one without counting them, they are still there and they still exist. It's a choice you have – be accurate or guess. Know or don't know. Would you rather wing things or know things? Have a think about that. Knowing how food contributes to fat loss is the one thing you have ignored for years and, in doing so, is the biggest factor as to why you believe that self-sabotaging was necessary. Being mindful of calories in those impulsive moments, when you get offered a biscuit at work or have a glass of champagne at a birthday party, will influence what happens next!

Calories offer perspective and help prevent self-sabotage. It's not about having the exact amount of calories in your lunch, it's just knowing that you're roughly having similar amounts but using different foods that in that moment were convenient.

what foods are good and bad for fat loss?

We get asked this every single day. What are the best foods for fat loss? Which foods aren't good for fat loss? Well, hopefully you're starting to realise there is no such thing as good or bad foods. Really the only way to categorise them, other than foods you like and foods you don't, is based upon what we mentioned before, their **nutrient density**. Nutrient-dense foods are much more nourishing for our bodies and contain lots of vitamins and minerals. All that is very important for health, skin, teeth, sleep and appetite, but it will not determine you being in a negative energy balance, the calorie deficit needed to lose body fat.

What we are going through here is a myth-busting process. As part of that, food doesn't need to go under the microscope, it just needs to be discussed with some perspective. Without question, a diet rich in nutrient-dense foods is optimum, but what's more important is having a balanced approach and eating an abundance of different foods that are not seen as good or bad. That could look like a mixture of salads and smoothies, a takeaway and a shop-bought sandwich. It's not an all-or-nothing approach, it's making sure you're mindful of the healthy stuff but are also able to enjoy the less healthy stuff, because, well, it's tasty!

Putting foods into categories of good or bad is a recipe for disaster. What's worse is that fad diets don't categorise based on nutrient density either, instead they come up with some gimmick suggesting certain foods work for fat loss better than others. We're sure you've followed fad diets that have removed some food groups completely, for example, low carb diets, thus demonising foods that contain heaps of vitamins and minerals like potatoes, pulses, wholegrains and fruit.

The main way that eating certain types of foods can influence fat loss is from a mental perspective, to make things more comfortable and enjoyable. So, choosing foods that you like and that you can stick with long term means consistent results.

Often when this whole 'good versus bad food' stigma causes problems it's in those unexpected moments where you must react quickly. Like when you forget to set your alarm and don't have time for your usual breakfast, or when you forget your lunch for work. You need to quickly make a choice and more often than not that choice is seen as being a bad one.

Let's say you're following a fad diet with no focus on calories at all. You just prepare food based on a restrictive list of ingredients you've been told you must follow, i.e. 'good' food. You get to work and realise you left lunch in the fridge, so what do you do? You're miles from home so can't pop back for it and you're hungry. The options available to you don't change based on understanding fat loss or not, but your perspective will. How you feel in that moment and how the rest of your day will pan out as a result of what you do. So you pop to the shops and you grab a meal deal (full of anxiety, no doubt) and can only think about this being a bad choice.

Let's change what you know for a moment. Imagine you were calorie-aware and knew your lunch equated to 500 calories. Think about how informed your decision-making process would be, how much more comfortable and relaxed you'd be. The sandwich as part of the meal deal was 375 calories, the crisps were 150 calories and the Diet Coke – nothing. You see, knowledge is power, and that's what fad diets don't want you to have. Power over them to say well, actually I don't like eating in this way and I know I don't have to, so I'll do things my way.

Calories offer perspective and help to prevent self-sabotage. It's not about having the exact amount as contained in your lunch, it's just knowing that you are roughly having similar amounts but using different foods in that moment.

feeling guilty

Sadly, at that time of self-sabotage, you didn't have the perspective of calories in versus calories out, which meant your focus was on going off plan with food that was bad. So you don't recap on the months of physical progress you've made, how you've become better at cooking, more organised and productive. You have tunnel vision and all you can worry about is that off-plan meal. If self-sabotage is the number one reason why people don't succeed on a fad diet, then feeling guilty is the number one emotion that sparks self-sabotage in the first place. The key here is to prevent that emotion from happening.

What is the instinctive thing we all try to do when we do something wrong? We try to correct it! Damage control, as it's known in the fad dieting world, can range from doing things like reducing the size of your dinner, doing an extra workout or skipping a meal altogether. In some cases, people won't eat for twenty-four hours. We've seen and experienced it all and we are sure you have been there. Can you think of the most drastic thing you did to try and counteract going off plan? YOU. HAVE. DONE. NOTHING. WRONG . . . #itsfine.

Just like eating one bowl of salad will not make someone skinny, eating one shop-bought sandwich, a chocolate bar or a packet of crisps will not make you morbidly obese. These circumstances will always happen, and eventually, through overcoming one episode, then another and another, you'll see results still happen and you will realise that you didn't need to worry or feel guilty at all. We actually want everyone to go through these moments as part of the plan, as it's one of the most important parts of what we do and what you need to experience. And best of all, it's all part of being on plan.

On a final note, when it comes to this type of situation and being mindful of calories, we want to let you into a little secret that not many people really know . . . You don't have to be in a calorie deficit every day to lose weight. You really don't. So, with that in mind, if you're thinking, what if the calories aren't the same as what I had planned? Then you'll now know #itsfine. During these situations, some of you will have managed in the past to shake yourself and move forward that day without feeling terrible and throwing in the towel, only to be met by the most ruthless problem of all . . . the following day's weigh-in.

the weight loss lottery

Honestly, we could write an entire book based purely on weighing yourself correctly. But for now, let's focus on doing it as part of your process of justification. We've already said we are pro-scales, but only as a very small part of the measuring process done correctly, not as a method to determine how much fat you gained from eating something different the day before.

Did you know that of everything that's done as part of fad diet culture, the hardest thing for us to move people away from is weighing themselves. It's like an addiction, and the idea of not doing it is quite daunting, isn't it? We appreciate habits are hard to break, especially ones you've been doing for years, but it's important to take small steps that will eventually add up to big changes. This is one of them.

The trouble is that most people who weigh in after going 'off plan' usually weigh in frequently and, more often than not, did so the day before as well. So there is an immediate comparison that can be made. A snapshot in time that shows nothing relevant of the day before. Have you ever had a blood test that's covered things like cholesterol and blood sugar, for example? Most people at some point in their lives will have done and, quite often, depending on you and your lifestyle, the results (as part of this snapshot in time) can indicate your need to improve your overall health. In other words, become more active, reduce your intake of salt and saturated fats and be mindful of what you eat in general. So you run with that advice and make an effort to improve yourself without a second thought, but you don't get a blood test every day or every week to measure your progress, do you? You don't throw in the towel because one day you didn't go to the gym, you just accept in any one week that you are taking positive steps forwards. But when it comes to weight, it's a daily obsessive ritual that you feel you must do.

The problem you face in this scenario is that the day before (which followed a few weeks of being on a restrictive plan) you weighed in at X, which was as a result of eating small portions of food, no doubt lower in sugar and salt, and kept everything pretty stable. But now, due to a quite substantial upscale of meal size and increase in carb intake, your body has chosen to behave a little differently. You have not gained any fat, but just a little bit of extra weight in the form of water. However, you don't think about any of this, you might not even know about this, you're just ready to gamble and play the weight loss lottery which, like any game, has no guaranteed win.

What happens next? You hop on the scales and, sure enough, it's a gain! That takes any positivity you had about your progress and turns it on its head. Let's just hope it wasn't a Friday, because then the entire weekend is up for grabs and the blowout will be even more intense.

But that little tiny number has now determined the outcome for you, because the number one goal for any fad diet is weight loss on the scales and so a gain is not acceptable. At this point, you feel eating whatever you want is a suitable punishment for going off plan. It's self-sabotage at its worse and it's you punishing yourself for nothing. You won't have gained a gram of body fat, let alone a pound. It's worth bearing in mind that to gain 1lb of body fat requires you to eat around 3,500 calories (at least) over the amount you need in any one day to maintain your body weight. So, all in all, taking into account what you now know about calories and the energy also required to digest and metabolise food (yes, that uses energy as well), you will have needed perhaps 5,000 calories in food just to gain 1lb. Now you've stepped on the scales, and it's come back with a gain of 3lbs! Impossible in this scenario.

In these moments, which will form part of the new journey as you adjust to saying #itsfine, you must distance yourself from the scales. They will never show the reality of what's going on in your body and do not control your life anymore.

The key take home is that, although the reasons for you self-sabotaging aren't valid, the emotional connection to these situations and obstacles are very real. Even when you truly understand there is a much healthier way to react, you still need to anticipate the potential obstacles as part of your new journey.

It's a lot easier to stick to a new way of thinking when the conditions are just right, but it's important to be aware that no journey is perfect. If you want to prevent self-sabotage for good, be prepared to go through a few uncomfortable experiences at the start. Don't worry though, it's all part of saying #itsfine and, even if you have had a wobble, it's all on plan.

Finally, readdress your values, because diets have a nasty habit of changing them to keep you signed up to their way of thinking and measuring success. Make sure they determine your priorities and represent a true measure of how your journey is going, because when the things that you do don't align with your personal values, that's when things feel wrong or bad and create feelings of guilt. What you should most value is you and your health.

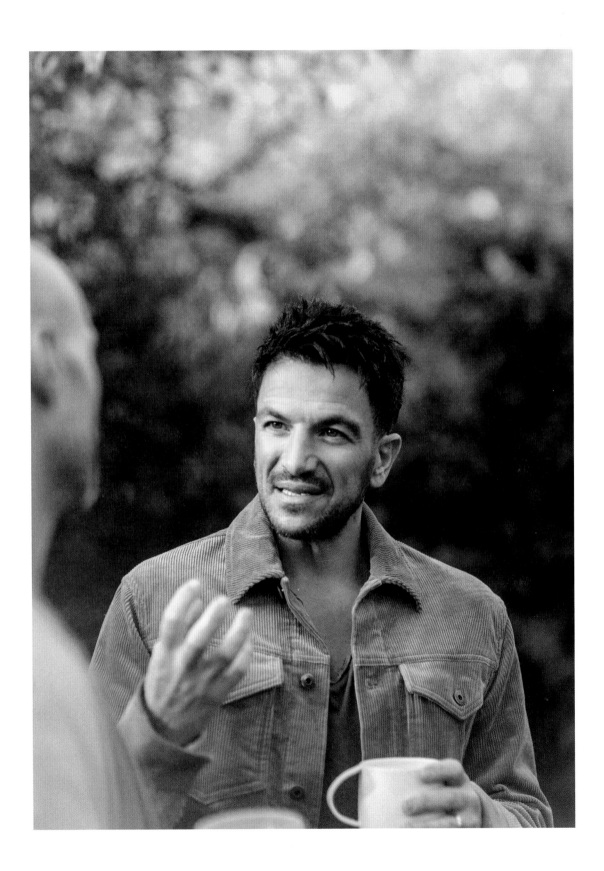

Chapter 4

EXPOSING
FAD DIETS

the truth just isn't sexy, is it? honesty just doesn't sell . . .

It's very important that you come to terms with the fad diets you have done and the false promises and 'facts' they have sold you. To achieve this, we wanted to put some of the most popular ones under the microscope, as well as expose the ones that fall under the radar and appear to be something 'new' and/or 'different', which leads you to believe they could be just the answer.

To us, anything that does not place an emphasis on portion control, nutrition and lifestyle is what is known as a fad diet. We have mentioned that we pride ourselves on being those things that diets are not, and that is transparent, honest and truly tailored to the individual. Anything that restricts food groups, sets you on a rigid plan with a strict formula, with an emphasis only on weight within a certain time period, is a fad diet. Another good way to get some clarity on whether you have followed a fad diet or not is that you should never be doing something that you either can't or don't like doing. This not only goes for food, but also for routine, structure and type of exercise. So how on earth can something not have been created sooner when the problems are so obvious?

We remember conceptualising #itsfine and speaking to various people who all unanimously said, 'But what makes you unique and how are you going to market yourself against all those giant powerhouses?' While other businesses search for that gimmick, that hook, that new magic formula, shake or pill, we don't. We understand that the obesity epidemic does not need a quick fix, a promise of fast results, or yet another plan that claims to bypass the laws of science, specifically calories in versus calories out. We know that often the reason you haven't gone for an evidence-based approach in the first place is because it seems, well, a bit bland and long-winded. Therefore, the uphill battle for us to get people started within one of the most competitive marketplaces in the world is redefining what a weight loss journey looks like.

Now picture this. If we went toe to toe on a marketing campaign with a fad diet, on the face of it, we would not appear as attractive. Which one would you typically go for?

Get in the shape of your life in 30 days and be beach-ready in no time!

Learn how to eat the foods you love over a year using weekly calories, embarking on a journey of trial and error that will eventually enable you to get sustained long-term results.

Don't worry, we won't take it personally, because for us at #itsfine, we would rather help fewer people and do it correctly for the long term, than help millions achieve a short-term weight loss that can't be sustained. The key to success is down to the value it adds to people's lives and the positive impact it will have long term. Deep down, if you really think about it, all your goals are long term. It's just that the promise of something happening quickly is attractive and you will deal with the aftermath of struggling to sustain it later on.

Here's one for you . . . a staggering 98 per cent of people we have worked with online over twelve years come to us from a background of failing on a fad diet. We hear about their different stories, problems and situations, but they are all suffering from the same group of terrible, restrictive and generic fad diet plans.

We always say when embarking on a weight loss journey, that you need to be the engineer and not the customer. That may sound daunting and complex, but rest assured, it's not. You feel that way because you don't know anything other than what you've been roped into believing. Fad diets use this to their advantage by presenting something that on the surface is very simple, but they don't supply you with a warranty. So, when the inevitable happens and it breaks down (which of course it will, due to its shoddy design), when you come across those obstacles, you won't have the understanding to address the cause of the problem.

Fad diets believe that the way you get people to start, and keep them going, is a result of what happens in the first week or two. In other words, they experience a rapid drop on the scales, which in turn keeps them excited and motivated so they stick to the diet. This could not be further from the truth and actually it's what happens in the first four to twelve weeks that sets you up for life. Think of it in terms of a career. You would never start a job expecting to become the CEO of a company in a matter of weeks. You first need to learn the ropes and go through the ups and downs of the job before it starts to get comfortable. You can then do the job in your sleep, at which point you get offered a promotion. That promotion, just like with a new goal, means you making adjustments, learning something new, being more hands-on, so after some time, that new role becomes second nature. But instead, you rush into a position you aren't ready for, with hours that don't suit you, with day-to-day tasks you can't keep up with and then you resign.

Instead, know that in the future you will achieve that role, that goal of becoming CEO, but accept that it won't happen overnight. The trick is to ignore all that white noise telling you the overwhelming norm is that fat loss should be fast, quick and easy, and then when it isn't, you quit.

what's under the bonnet

By now you're starting to realise that fat loss only occurs when you're in a negative energy balance, when you're eating less food (energy) than your body needs. If you took every single success story from every fad diet on earth and looked at their calorie consumption, they would all have been in a calorie deficit. We call these people the lucky ones, because they winged it and, as a result of what they ate and how active they were, they got into a calorie deficit. Those who were not successful (by successful, we mean the number on the scales went down) were not so lucky and either ended up eating more food than their body needed or just the right amount to sustain their body weight. So, by lifting the bonnet, the engine in all these cases will look the same, but what fad diets do is try to make the car look sexy, go faster and seem more comfortable.

We aren't here to name and shame. What we want to do though is break down the popular ways you are sold the dream of weight loss and lead that all back to biology, the fact you ate less or more food than your body needed. Some or most of these you will be aware of, whereas others may come as a complete surprise, especially the newer methods.

very low calorie diets (vlcds)

This is a good one to start with because, on the face of it, it at least recognises portion control as a method for fat loss. This type of diet was put in place in the 1970s, initially as a rapid weight loss programme whereby calories were severely restricted. These diets mainly targeted those who needed to lose weight quickly because of severe health issues that came about as a result of being super-morbidly obese, often being bedbound.

There are many factors at play, such as disease and mobility problems, which cause people to be in this situation. However, in very many cases, it's due to a substantial overconsumption of calories. When you go from consuming such a large amount of food, likely to be over 5,000 calories per day, then slash that to say 800–1,000 calories a day, your body is going to do the only thing it has been designed to do and it will get its energy requirements from elsewhere . . . body fat.

Having been in this industry for a while now, we have actually seen some people (a tiny, tiny percentage) make long-term progress with VLCDs. That success came only because of a unique mindset that allowed them to remain focused and motivated, despite feeling very hungry all day, every day. This was coupled with an ability to switch themselves over to a higher number of calories progressively when their goal was reached, without slipping back into old ways. They would also have had the combined assistance of specialists and doctors to support and counsel them, which would have helped massively. We can't express how rare that is, but we believe at least having an understanding of the concept of eating less (regardless of what that is) gave them a transparent starting point and frame of reference.

The problem we face with these VLCDs is that they are much more accessible to the general public now and come in the form of a microwave meal or a shake. These, alongside the promise of rapid weight loss, come with the convenience of not needing to cook and being easy to carry around. Some see these as a good strategy for getting ready for a holiday or a wedding, whereas others, with no experience of calories at all, see them as a good starting point.

There is a saying we put to everyone who is on a diet: 'Can you see yourself doing what you're doing now five years down the line and being happy?' And that means eating (and also drinking) less than a five-year-old child forever. We don't think so.

These commercial VLCDs are insensitive to building a long-term calorie adjustment plan for you, one that gives you a range to move down from. Instead, your calories are set so low, often to breaking point in terms of your hunger and energy levels, that when the weight loss stops you feel stuck. This won't happen overnight, of course, as it takes a lot longer than you think for your body to hit a plateau and therefore need your calories to be reassessed. In reality, it's often not down to the calories at all, but the way you weigh yourself or the fact that you haven't remained consistently on a VLCD for long enough. But let's just say you have remained on it consistently for six months (somehow) and fat loss has stopped. What do you do? Well, ideally, you'd look at increasing output, in other words movement and activity. But you're on a VLCD so your primary focus is calories, therefore, you try to drop them down and end up on 600 calories a day, or less! Not only is this going to put a huge amount of pressure on things like your hormones, vital oragns and immune system, it's going to make you miserable to the point where you have dropped them so low you either faint or quit.

The industry has taken something that was only used in severe and urgent medical cases, with people whose lives were in danger, and packaged that up for the rest of the world.

When looking at your overall portion sizes and calorie requirements, it's never a one-size-fits-all approach. The golden rule? Always start as high as possible, eating as much food as possible. We find that people we've worked with who are coming off a VLCD can lose weight on double, if not triple, the number of calories they were on, we just took the time to find that out for them. So, calories, yes, a good starting point, but a drastically low amount, no.

magical foods

If there was ever a principle that, on the face of it, ignored calories completely, yet solely relied on you being in a calorie deficit, it's this one! Not only that, it takes the premise of portion control and calories in versus calories out (1+1 = 2, for example) and turns it into an equation that you try to solve, yet has no correct answer. Because it's wrong.

Imagine being able to eat as much of certain foods as you like and somehow not put on weight. In fact, being able to lose it! But on the flip side, irrelevant of calories, there are some foods that make you put on weight much more easily, so you have to stay away from them. Just to make things even more bizarre, combining and/or cooking or not cooking foods (eating them raw), will also have a bearing on how you lose or gain weight.

Let's be clear about something from the get-go here. An overconsumption of the good stuff, the most nutrient-dense foods on the planet, will still result in fat gain. The same goes for an under-consumption of bad stuff, which will result in fat loss.

For these methods to be initially successful, it very much depends on the person doing it fitting into a very small group of people who enjoy a certain type of food(s) and dislike others. What they don't seem to care about is that we are all very different. Not only do our bodies have totally different needs, but our appetites are also very different, not to mention our relationships with food.

This really is like rolling a dice here, it's just a game of chance, which is why you will see some people do well but the vast majority failing.

Firstly, let's meet Becky. Becky had a good upbringing around food. Her parents made sure she ate a balanced diet and, as a result, she enjoys a variety of different fruits and vegetables, more so than say meat, fish and poultry. Becky isn't a fan of processed foods and doesn't have a huge appetite. Although her relationship with food at this point is OK, she has hit her forties and feels that she isn't looking how she would like, making her lack a bit of confidence.

Now, let's meet Sarah. Sarah didn't have the best upbringing around food. She had lots of siblings, busy parents and food was much more about convenience. Her diet consisted mainly of beige foods thrown in the microwave or oven for 20 minutes, with a range of 'junk food' always available. She loves pasta, red meat and curries and has a large appetite, which has led her to put on a lot of unwanted fat. The thought of having a piece of fruit when hungry or tucking into a salad is just not appealing to her.

Who do you think would have done well with these magical food diets then? Becky or Sarah?

Well Becky mainly stuck to salads, fruit and vegetables, which she enjoyed. Being able to eat as much veg as she fancied was great and she'd often find it didn't leave much room on the plate for other things. So, she would add a piece of fish to her meals at various points of the week. She could eat as much fish as she liked, but people don't tend to gorge themselves on fish, do they? Funny that. Despite not being a massive fan of processed foods, treats and takeaways, she did often enjoy them in the past with friends and family. However, she now found herself thinking about them a lot more since they became limited or were seen as 'bad'. Becky lost weight and actually managed to sustain it by creating meals based on the type and amount of food that suited her. However, her relationship with food had got worse as she was now conditioned to see food as being 'good' or 'bad'. We bet it will only be a matter of time before Becky slips into feelings of guilt when she finally decides she is allowed to eat that slice of cake or have that meal out.

Sarah on the other hand lost the plot. After all, being able to eat as much of the food she personally enjoyed was what attracted her to this method of losing weight. She enjoyed huge piles of chicken curries, potato wedges with steaks and as many eggs as she could fit in. She stayed clear of fruit and veg, of course, as she wasn't a fan. Some days she would actually not eat anything until the evening, then make her meal using all the 'bad' stuff she was allowed while still being 'on plan'. This didn't work well for her, as once she got a taste for it, she would want more so would give in to temptation, often over the weekend, and say she'd restart on Monday eating as much of what was 'on plan' as possible, because she could. Sarah's relationship with food took a turn for the worse and she felt like something was wrong with her. 'It's worked for Becky', she thought, 'who's doing the same plan, so surely I must have done something wrong as I am actually putting on weight'.

Both Becky and Sarah are in a bad place now. However, from a weight loss perspective, Sarah seems to be struggling the most. There are no biologically magic foods out there that make fat vanish better than others, just like there are no foods out there that make it worse. You may well have experienced a fad diet like this and we hope you realise just how lucky you have to be to have long-term success using these methods.

low carb diets

Here we go again with yet another concept that uses a calorie deficit to lose weight but attributes its results to another gimmick. The claim is that, by reducing your carbohydrate intake, you will help your body burn fat instead of sugar for energy. In other words, let's remove a large food group almost entirely, so that you eat less and lose weight. Now, we are focusing on re-education here and perspective, not biochemistry and the negative effects certain types of carbohydrates can have on things like diabetes. Rightly so, because these fad diets don't talk about any of that, their primary focus is on you losing weight and it's the weight side of it that gets people excited, especially in the first week.

We have already said about how, when carbohydrates are consumed through food, the body stores any surplus as energy in the muscles before it becomes the wobbly stuff. When you aren't eating and haven't eaten for a while, your body will start tapping into those energy reserves and, in turn, deplete them from your system, along with the water that is used to store them in the first place. This is all very normal stuff, so you eat a meal again containing carbohydrates and the cycle continues as it's meant to, which is great.

But what happens when you eat meals with almost no carbohydrates in them at all? Well, without eating carbs, you aren't going to be storing energy from them and, with that, no water. So that means those stored energy reserves are used, but not topped back up, and your body weight (but not body fat) initially will drop significantly as a result. Depending on your size and muscle mass, this could be as much as a few kilograms. That's the first thing you will notice on the scales and boy, are you happy! However, even if you were eating at your maintenance level calories, even in a small surplus, you would still likely see a drop in the scales during the first weigh-in. This is a great example of why dropping or gaining weight is not always attributed to dropping or gaining body fat.

In the following weeks, things can slow but may still head in the right direction for you. Most of the time that's because you're in a large calorie deficit due to all your favourite foods being removed, leaving you with a small choice of fat and protein-rich ingredients you aren't a fan of, so won't over-consume.

For fat loss, this type of restrictive method is often very unhealthy, very unpleasant and extremely unsociable. Not only are things like chocolate, cakes and sweets demonised, so are nutrient-dense foods packed full of fibre like wholegrains, pasta, pulses and fruits.

We are massive advocates of everyone being able to eat what they enjoy as part of a balanced healthy diet, and if you aren't a huge fan of carbohydrate-rich foods then #itsfine. Our issue comes when you're advised to follow a low-carb plan that leaves you feeling tired, deprived and unhappy, eating foods you hate. All that fad diet did was remove a huge food group, which in turn made you eat less and weigh less due to the body not doing what it's fundamentally designed to do, that being the storage and utilisation of energy.

intermittent fasting (if)

Right then, skipping a meal now has a title! Not only that, it's also incredible for fat loss. But let's look at the science behind that. Taking say, 500 calories out of your day, every day, for a week, would result in losing fat. Honestly, being laid out like that, transparently, as a way of eating less and creating a calorie deficit, we don't have an issue.

But that's not how it's marketed, which means you aren't able to make an informed decision. We've got to admit, it takes a real genius to be able to commercialise skipping breakfast or not eating for a day or two by simply adding in the word 'intermittent'. What we want to know is, what would have been wrong with calling it say:

- **Infrequent eating**
- **Occasional dining**
- **Periodic consumption**
- **Meal skipping**

From our recollection, intermittent fasting became mainstream around ten years ago and different variations of it have been popping up year after year ever since.

This style of consuming meals means you only eat during a specific time, increasing your fasting window and decreasing your eating window. The top three ways of doing this are:

1. Finish eating in the evening one day, then start again at lunchtime the next day with a six-to-eight hour eating window.

2. An entire 24-hour fast.

3. The extremely odd version where you eat many more calories than normal for 80 per cent of the week and then spend a couple of days eating much fewer calories, which, of course, isn't fasting.

What are the claims of intermittent fasting then? Fasting for ten to sixteen hours or longer can improve blood sugar balance, reduce inflammation and improve brain function. They then come in with the weight loss claims, such as 'and it will cause the body to turn its fat stores into energy, which releases ketones into the bloodstream, which in turn results in fat loss'.

Fasting has been investigated for decades now for its unique health benefits, and no doubt there probably are some. But trying to suggest it's optimum for fat loss and convincing people it's the answer to all their problems just isn't right. Especially as there isn't any emphasis on portion control whatsoever. And guess what? Have you ever met anyone doing any form of intermittent fasting who ate in a calorie surplus and lost body fat consistently? Of course not, because it's impossible.

There are a whole host of things you do at different times in life because they suit your lifestyle. You could get ten people in a room and every one of them will do it differently. Your perspective of that could be they're doing it 'intermittently', with the result being the same for all of you. For example, you may work longer hours in one go than your friend does, because that's the nature of your shift work. You then, in turn, have a longer period of time off work. They do a standard nine-to-five day and take the weekend off. Which one of them is doing 'intermittent' work? Have you ever used that phrase in your life?

What about people who have different sleeping routines, do they 'intermittent' sleep? Of course not. Remarkable how fad diets get away with things, isn't it?!

Everything has to have a name or a gimmick in the world of fad diets, otherwise you wouldn't buy into them. Honesty and transparency just doesn't sell, right? But fasting for weight loss really isn't a thing, it's merely an eating strategy that gets presented to you and either suits you or doesn't.

If you don't want breakfast, #itsfine. If you do, then #itsfine. If eating two meals instead of three suits you, #itsfine. If not eating for a day sometimes suits you, #itsfine. If you don't feel hungry for half the day and it doesn't affect your sleep, energy levels, work rate, fitness and mood, then crack on and do it. We have a substantial number of people using our app that miss out snacks and meals on certain days due to their shift work, lifestyle and appetite and we tell them #itsfine. But they don't give it a name or do it because it's magic, it's just part of what suits their lifestyle.

For you and your journey, do not think that meal frequency is advantageous for physical fat loss, because it's not. Some people thrive on the conventional approach of three meals a day, plus a snack mid-morning and mid-afternoon. Whereas for others, they just don't get hungry in the morning. There is no right or wrong. Removing a meal or a snack can be a very useful tool, but in the grand scheme of things, it's just a method of managing portion control and if that's not right for you, then you don't need to do it.

'not quite' intuitive eating

First of all, the premise behind intuitive eating is great and not something we have an issue with. However, we do have a problem with the timing of when it's introduced and how it's promoted as an 'anti-diet', then, when purchased, it's nothing more than a guided approach on how to consume food.

In a nutshell, intuitive eating is about making peace with food (which we love) and eating what feels right for you until you're full, by listening to your body and its hunger cues. Tapping into your natural ability to tell yourself when you're either hungry or satisfied. Not only that, you also let go of the idea that you need to lose weight.

When you're conscious that you want to lose weight, but have a negative relationship with food as well as having binge or emotional eating tendencies, you're far from being ready for the true meaning of this approach or for doing anything around food intuitively. Being able to eat intuitively is an advanced technique that takes years of conditioning. You may never achieve it, simply because food for you will always have some conscious purpose, but that's OK. Intuitive eating means reaching decisions quickly with food based on an automatic subconscious thought process, not a reflective one that considers other possibilities, ingredients, etc. However, instead of offering this to the correct type of person as a real, long-term approach, we are now seeing this method being used as a marketing tool to get you to sign up to something that couldn't be further from behaving intuitively.

There is a scary new wave of fad diets that place a sole emphasis on mindful eating, where it's all about psychology and not tracking your food intake, miraculously still achieving weight loss. These guys are very sneaky, as they initially appear to be a long way away from a fad diet. Some of you may have signed up to them online. They're usually exceptionally expensive and offer you a personal therapist as part of the process. You will undergo an extensive evaluation with dozens of unusual questions about your life and you will, at the end of it, receive a programme. But guess what that programme entails? A recipe/food guide that, when things don't work, they back up with further information on portion control and, dare we say it, calories. This is as far away from an intuitive way of behaving around food as you can get, but they suck you in. The only saving grace is that your therapist will eventually talk to you about food and how much you should be eating, but you didn't sign up for that, did you?

so, it was calories all along then!

Yep, that's right. Whether they choose to admit it or not, the only way the weight loss happens is through portion control and a calorie deficit. A calorie deficit will happen because you planned it, or because you fluked it, but either way, that's why you lost body fat.

We believe the best way to make peace with food is to understand it. Not the complex science of macronutrients, digestion and metabolism, just the basics we've already shown you that had been hidden from you.

In the next chapter, we introduce you to a new, simplified way of managing your calories that doesn't rely on checking them day to day, but instead week to week. It's time now to get acquainted with weekly portion control and see how flexible it really is.

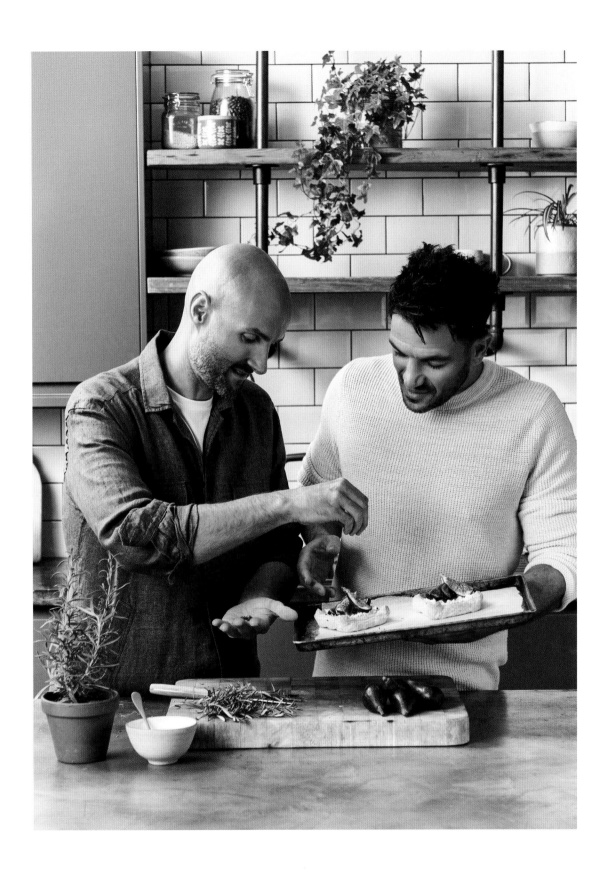

Chapter 5

MAKING FRIENDS WITH PORTION CONTROL

what fad diets don't want you to know

For most of you, before reading this book, you probably wouldn't have had a good understanding of calories, how they work and their importance as a measure of energy balance, which in turn results in fat loss. Even though you're aware of this now, you need to get to grips with what you do with that information and how you apply it to your life.

The initial problem with counting calories is people's perception of what's involved, with words being thrown around like obsessive, complex and stressful. We don't agree and prefer to use words like accurate, responsible and useful.

The funny thing is that most people with that negative mentality have been taught it through fad diet culture. But in many other areas of their lives, they do things that can be seen as contradicting what put them off calories in the first place. For example, you take an inaccurate measurement of what's happening with fat loss in the form of the bathroom scales and weigh yourself obsessively every day. That number is used to determine how well you're doing. All the while signed up to a fad diet that you will quite happily follow based on using a complex formula you must stick to religiously each day, but one that actually has no accuracy behind it. So, in essence, you're behaving in the exact way that your negative perception of calories is based upon; this same perception is the reason you have chosen not to be mindful of them.

Understanding what's really going on is the ultimate key to breaking people away from a life of calorie-absent fad diets, rescuing you from your core factual beliefs around food and showing you the light. There are lots of people out there trying to help you with good intentions, pulling you as far away from portion control as possible, focusing on introducing you to a wider range of foods and habits. But unless you fully believe in something and understand it, you will second-guess everything you do, because you're so used to what you have done in the past, which will always be your frame of reference.

Now we've established that what you were attracted to in the past and what you have done for years was in fact tracking something, albeit inaccurately. But let's look at another completely acceptable and normal way of keeping track of an important part of your life . . . your finances.

For some of you reading this, being able to access information about how you're saving and spending your money has always been attainable. However, for many of you, you'll remember the inconvenience of either having to check a statement at a cash machine or queue up at lunchtime to get the cashier to print one. Not only that, the surprise of the balance was not always what you expected!

In the banking industry, being able to suddenly access your account online was revolutionary and welcomed by many people. I'm sure it contributed massively in a positive way to helping you manage your money. Portion control does just that, except your currency is food. Just imagine being criticised for managing your finances, accurately spending your money wisely and not going overdrawn. As if anyone is going to do that and, even if they did, it would usually be because somebody is envious of the good habits and behavioural traits that you have, wishing they were like you, well informed and confident. You'll find this a lot in the world of dieting as well.

This is a good frame of reference and comparison, so let's keep this analogy of spending and saving through online banking at the front of our minds as we move forward. Another important point to make is that you do not need to check your finances every day to be good at managing them. Nor do you need to reflect on every single transaction, as your running balance is often the only indication you need to know you're heading in the right direction. But that said, having the option to understand each transaction (what's going on) has got to be useful, right?

Fad diets aren't capable of facilitating the management of your money correctly. Instead of using an accurate measurement of your country's currency, they decide to call it something else and have it behave quite differently, assuring you it's better that way. Imagine if we told you that you could spend more money than you earn or have in your bank and it would have no bearing at all on your finances. No repercussions, no penalties and actually you should just accept it and move on positively. Well, you're not going believe that are you? But at one point with your previous fad diet, you did.

Of course, if you were one of those people like so many others that really decided to go for it and went on a spending spree, you'd have been subject to some hefty charges in the future, reflected not on your account on your phone, but on your bathroom scales. When you then question what's happened, they don't show you the transactions in your currency, but instead in another. The longer you spend in this way, the harder it is to see how and why things are happening.

In the UK's case, a pound is a pound. Regardless of how you spend it, be that knowingly and mindfully, or going for it without a care in the world 'hoping' you remain in credit or within your balance. If that pound gets spent at a different time of day, in a different shop, a different country or among other transactions, it's still going to equate to the same thing.

We have been honest about this from the start and part of your journey with #itsfine will involve ups and downs and obstacles that will require your attention. Like when your card is declined due to a little overspending perhaps. Except we will bring it to your attention and show you where improvements can be made. You see the only time these obstacles become a problem is when you go back and forth trying to do the same thing, whereas the reality is to adjust something very minor and then overcome it quickly. Knowledge really is power for you here and by reassuring you from the get-go that something like a fat loss plateau is merely an inevitable point in your journey, we give you the answers and guidance to either see it's nothing at all, or work out how to adjust it so you'll have nothing to worry about. If you can't accurately reflect on and understand what got you to a certain point, it's extremely hard to get past that. It's in these moments where portion control and calories are used to make well-informed, practical decisions.

So, to summarise, having an understanding of what you're earning against what you're spending is great. But at the same time, being successful with managing your balance doesn't mean checking it every single day, and for the vast majority of you who are managing your finances well, you can relate to this and feel comfortable knowing that actually achieving weight loss can work in the same way.

weekly calories: the best-kept secret that everyone 'not' on a diet does . . .

We'd like to draw your attention back to what we believe deep down is your overriding goal. To feel and behave 'normally' around food, just like those around you seem to do. Be they friends, family members or colleagues, you want to be like them. More than once you've asked yourself: How do they do it? How can they be like that, always looking the same and yet seeming to eat anything they like? Well, guess what, we know . . .

Let's first talk about what you think is going on. The big one is 'they must just have a really fast metabolism'. How many times have you thought that and then concluded that yours must be slow, causing you to do very drastic things? Let's not dismiss this completely, because some people do have very good genes and can consume more food than others. But, in our experience, it's your perception of what they are doing that is all off.

Doing something once doesn't define us. We are the sum total of what we do overall and consistently. As we touched on before, eating one bar of chocolate won't make you fat, just the same as one salad won't make you skinny. This is very relevant here because normally when you see this friend, family member or colleague, it's either during social events or at a set time each day, at work, for example, and this is just a snapshot into how they live their life and how they eat.

Let's focus on a work colleague for now, Laura. Some days when Laura gets in she is drinking the leftovers of a drive-through cappuccino. Some mornings she has some biscuits with a cup of tea, and you'd swear it had sugar in it. At lunch, she always pops to the supermarket and brings back a sandwich, a bag of crisps and a bar of chocolate. Sometimes mid-afternoon you even see her eating another biscuit or two with her cuppa! She comes in the following week talking about the amazing takeaway she and the family enjoyed at the weekend! In your mind, you're looking at someone who looks great but appears to be able to eat a ton of food, all of which is off limits for you; it's not fair! But it's what you're NOT seeing which is so important, and that's her balanced approach.

What Laura actually does is take her dog for a walk in the morning, the distance depends on if she got things ready for the kids the night before, but that walk can sometimes last an hour and that's a decent 5km. Laura likes to feel like she is doing something good for her body and, as a rule, likes to start her day off with a smoothie. She doesn't pay a huge amount of attention to the amounts of things, but it's full of fruit and vegetables with a splash or two of almond milk. Sometimes the mornings are just too hectic, though, so instead, on the way in, she grabs a nice coffee as a pick-me-up. On those days, she feels a little peckish in the morning, so she'll enjoy a biscuit or two. Her lunch is the staple of her day and remains consistent.

When Laura finishes work, she's often quite tired but still has a fair amount to do around the house with her kids, getting their dinner ready, etc., so sometimes she'll pinch a fish finger or two from the oven tray and then sit down in the evening and have something convenient to eat, which may just go in the microwave. The weekend is family time and one of the things they like to enjoy together is a Saturday night takeaway, usually a curry or a pizza. Laura sticks mainly to what she knows with a curry, having a main course with some rice and a few poppadoms, and if it's pizza, she shares one with her husband.

What you've got here is essentially a good relationship with food that over the course of any week has a bit of everything. There is routine and spontaneity, as well as some good habits. But what you thought Laura did versus what she actually does were two very different things. Day to day it's not the same. Some days she didn't eat breakfast at all, giving a bit of substance behind why she has tea and biscuits in the morning and comes in with a coffee. Laura also likes to keep active in the morning, no intense training session there but all movement is good. Her lunch is the staple of her day and is able to remain consistent. Could her food be more nutrient-dense? Well, yes, but a healthy mind is just as important, and let's not forget, she doesn't live on crisps and chocolate. Some evenings she can really end up just picking on bits or heating up leftovers like spag bol or a microwave meal, so this doesn't amount to much. When that weekend comes and Saturday arrives, it's not a case in Laura's mind that she has earned anything. That takeaway is just a regular thing she does to bring the family together. Food is and should be seen as happiness, you know.

Laura looks the way she does not because of her body being magic, but because when she gets to the end of an average week, she just happens to be either at maintenance level with her calories or in a small deficit. During the odd week here and there, she may even be in a calorie surplus, but #itsfine because, when your measurement of progress physically is over the long term not the short term, it's irrelevant.

People like this subconsciously live their lives based on weekly calories. So, while there is no magic here, there is a secret. It's just not something people with a good relationship with food are aware of, because it's habitual and something they don't even realise is happening. Balance is key and we believe the best way to get you there is to have an open and honest plan and show you how it all works, then build that into your week to become your very own Laura.

daily calories: a guide and a tool (but not an obsession)

When it comes to being mindful of your daily calorie intake, don't worry that if you're not then fat loss won't happen. Just like the nutrients you put in your body on one particular day will not determine how healthy you are, the calories you consume in a day will not have a huge impact on your long-term fat loss goals. This is what a lot of people who obsess about daily calorie counting just don't get. The culture of weighing yourself every day has a huge part to play in that, as you trust it as a method for monitoring body fat. What you get shown you see as being a direct by-product of what you did the day before, but that just isn't true.

Think of fat loss as a marriage. You wouldn't get a divorce just because you and your partner had an argument one day, would you? You wouldn't question if they are the one and if it's working just because one day was different to the other? It's a long-term commitment and everything can be ticking along just right, without you analysing everything that happened at the end of each day, checking that it all went perfectly . . .

Being mindful of your daily calories is useful for other reasons. Of course, when you have a target amount to work towards in a week, the easiest way to hit that is by dividing it by seven days and sticking to that. But life isn't that simple and we all live day to day in very different ways. We don't like to feel restricted either, and being able to be flexible in what we do is what we all prefer. Not only that, contrary to popular belief, you don't need to be in a calorie deficit every day to lose fat.

So, what are the benefits of knowing what you eat each day? Firstly, it's a great tool for planning. Planning allows you to see in advance the things that will help you to achieve your goals, as well as the things that can potentially cause problems. For example, you may start planning breakfast, lunch, dinner and a couple of snacks all in line with your appetite and then realise you're consuming way too much. Knowing what you're adding in each day will allow you to identify what's tipping you over. It could be something as simple as your snacks contributing to this quite significantly. In fact, you may not even feel like snacking most of the time, so you remove/reduce them and before you know it, you're sorted.

But the most important reason is that daily calories will provide you with a frame of reference when eating away from a meal plan. Let's just say you did a simple sum of dividing your weekly target by seven, and then spread that out over three meals per day, where you got to around 500 calories per meal. Although you may structure your week in a totally different way, it's a frame of reference for you that, on average, a meal could amount to that. This is going to offer insight for being spontaneous, changing your mind or planning something different due to circumstances. This isn't you going 'off plan' though, as that's impossible with #itsfine, but just being mindful and knowing that your choices, whatever the food may be, will not stir up feelings of guilt or worry. This is so important when building a positive relationship with food.

Let's look at three very different situations.

1. You had your lunch in the fridge at work, but a colleague suggested a bite to eat somewhere. Well, this is nice and simple because you're aware of the calories (500 calories) for each meal, so you can aim to hit the same based on the information at the place you're going to eat. If it's a little over or under, that doesn't matter at all, #itsfine. If you find it's significantly over, you can choose to not worry at all (remember a day different to the one before is no issue) or instead reduce/omit a snack or two that same day or the day after.

2. You woke up one day and decided you wanted something different, something from the supermarket. By having that number in your head, you can just pick things up and put together something in and around that 500-calorie mark.

3. You have to travel for work somewhere long haul and won't be able to reheat your food on the train. In this situation, you can combine all three 500-calorie meals and run with a total of 1,500 calories, then apply that to anything from the shops available to you, as all the information is there, nice and simple.

All real, very normal circumstances, but ones that would've been extremely stressful for you in the past. As we move you through your plan, you'll also come to realise that #itsfine on some days if you don't know the calories or choose not to use them at all, honestly #itsfine. When your focus throughout the week is just one target, everything becomes so much easier, but that doesn't mean there isn't value in understanding and seeing what's happening each day.

so what are my calories then?

Here is a summary of what our social media inbox looks like on a daily basis:

Please can you tell me how much I should eat?

How many calories should I be on?

How do I know what I should be eating each day?

What's the easiest way of knowing how many calories I can have?

There is a growing popularity for calorie calculators that supposedly give you a magic daily calorie number that you can stick to forever and lose weight – all with different formulas and therefore all with different amounts. We've already talked through how sticking rigidly to a daily calorie amount is not needed in order to lose body fat, but actually sticking to a single number as a target also isn't required. Think back to Laura, she didn't and nor will you need to. We are not even going to provide you with one magic number to stick to. What you will get from us is a flexible calorie range . . .

Think of every single calorie counter you have used in the past and try to remember the numbers you were given. Same height, same weight, same age and same gender were entered, but you got this, for example:

- 1,450 calories per day

- 1,365 calories per day

- 1,512 calories per day

- 1,319 calories per day

Which weekly, looked like this:

- 10,150 calories per week

- 9,555 calories per week

- 10,584 calories per week

- 9,233 calories per week

There is very little in it really, a difference of 1,351 calories per week, which per day amounts to a 3km walk or, per meal, roughly less than the calories contained in a boiled egg. The reality could easily be that for you, on the lower end of the calorie scale, you were in a deficit of 20 per cent, and at the higher end around 12 per cent. What's important here is that ANY calorie deficit you're in is going to result in some amount of fat loss, in other words, progress.

So, if we had to trust this information and give you a starting point, we'd say to aim for a weekly calorie range of between 9,200 and 10,600 calories. This is just an example, but it should already be making some sense and showing you how much easier a weekly range is as opposed to a strict daily target, and this is how saying #itsfine works.

In the next chapter, we will take you through how to initially work out your weekly calorie starting point, building into that other lifestyle factors, then give you a nice simple range to work with. Work with, not succeed with, because truly tailored nutrition is a journey of discovery, but it's fun and will eventually determine a range that will not only result in fat loss, but have you saying #itsfine to all the food you enjoy!

Chapter 6
TAILORED FLEXIBILITY

the formula

Here we go, guys, it's time to start building your own tailored meal plan. One that gives you complete flexibility over what you eat, when you eat and how you eat.

Remember, this is the starting point and we'll make sure we give you a complete guide on how to monitor and tweak things during this crucial first stage of your #itsfine plan. Based on your history and background with fad diets, you're going to find this challenging at times. Not in terms of hunger, but just coming to terms with how flexible this is, what you can eat and trying your best not to have a sneaky peak at your physical progress too early on. Basically, you'll be thinking it's too good to be true, but with #itsfine, it really is that good!

This will look a lot more complicated than it is, but it's also the key to you finding a plan that will work for you long term. When you work through it yourself, you will see that it really is pretty straightforward and all you need is a pen and paper, a calculator and five minutes. Five minutes to change your life, that's not bad!

The first step is where a generic approach starts and ends with us. It's a formula we have used over many years with thousands of people and it serves as a great starting point.

Men:

[(10 x weight in kg) + (6.25 x height in cm) - (5 x age in years) + 5] x 7

Women:

[(10 x weight in kg) + (6.25 x height in cm) - (5 x age in years) - 161] x 7

Now multiply the outcome from the relevant calculation by the relevant category below to get your weekly target.

Chair or bedbound (none or minimal activity): 0.875

Seated work with little to no movement (think desk-bound all day): 1

Seated work with regular movement but not strenuous (such as van drivers or warehouse staff): 1.1

Standing work (on your feet all day, for example, shop assistants): 1.225

Strenuous work or highly active (constantly moving, with physical activity): 1.4

You now have a mid-point for your calorie target, but to open up a flexible range, we take your mid-point and **multiply by 0.9** (for the least amount of calories you can consume i.e. the starting point of your range), then we **multiply by 1.1** (to give you the largest amount of calories you can consume i.e. the end of your range).

Let's give you an example. Providing you have all this information to hand, it will be done within five minutes:

Jane Smith

So the correct formula is:

$$[(10 \times \text{weight in kg}) + (6.25 \times \text{height in cm}) - (5 \times \text{age in years}) - 161] \times 7$$

Weight: 80kg, therefore 10 x 80 = 800

Height: 170cm, therefore 6.25 x 170 = 1,063

Age: 40, therefore 5 x 40 = 200

Female: therefore – 161

On the calculator, Jane would do 800 + 1,063 – 200 – 161 = 1,502

Weekly number is: 1,502 x 7 = 10,514

Jane is a waitress and spends most of her day on her feet, therefore
10,514 x 1.225 = 12,880

Weekly range lower end: 12,880 x 0.9 = 11,592, so let's call that 11,600

Weekly range higher end: 12,880 x 1.1 = 14,168, so let's call that 14,150

So, Jane would be able to consume between 11,600 and 14,150 calories
per week.

Now let's move on to the final stage: exercise. In other words, anything else you do outside of your normal day. This could be gym workouts, football training, running, or even a dog walk. Contrary to popular belief, the overall percentage of calories burned in any one week comes mainly from your day-to-day movement, not your exercise. That said, to get to the most accurate weekly range, it's worth investing in a smart watch to track your additional activity outside of your daily norm. In other words, anything else you do other than waking up, going to work, coming home and then going to bed.

For some of you there is a daily routine, so you can forecast that additional energy expenditure easily in advance.

For example, if Jane's range is between 11,600 and 14,150 calories per week but she walks the dog every day, which her smart watch records as 250 calories per walk (x 7 for the week equates to 1,750 calories), then her more accurate range would be between 13,350 and 15,900 calories per week. How flexible is that?!

Most smart watches will give you a daily calorie burn taking into account your total step count, or heart rate fluctuations, but forget all that, please. It's just what you select as exercise that counts.

Now that you have this new total, does it mean you must eat 15,900 calories a week? No, it just means if you want to #itsfine. Furthermore, when using a weekly strategy, if the dog walk didn't happen one day, or you walked much further and burnt more calories in one walk, you can just adjust the total. Let's not forget though that within a range of calories, regardless of if it's the low end or the higher end, you're still in a deficit. So if you forget and don't want to make that adjustment, it literally doesn't matter as we don't have you living for a strict single number. #itsfine and there is no need to get obsessive.

There we have it, or at least Jane does in this example. Look at that – 13,350 to 15,900. How much easier is it having one flexible target for the week rather than seven strict ones?

One point on the whole smart watch accuracy front – don't cross over on devices and question which one is more accurate. Just pick one, and if you remain consistent, only refer to its estimate moving forward; #itsfine.

your lifestyle: a structure that suits you

This is what sets us apart from every fad diet you have ever done and makes us a truly tailored plan.

It's never really just the food you've eaten in the past that's made you miserable and caused you to throw in the towel. It's more about the fact that it just didn't work for your lifestyle.

The great news is that with #itsfine you'll find the food delicious and the way you eat it perfect. Why? Well, because you decide. With freedom of choice comes the first step, which is really discovering who you are and what works for you week on week. Here's a little stat for you. We haven't worked with a single person we know of who does the same thing months down the line that they did on day one. We don't mean the food specifically, but more the structure.

Building a lifelong strategy that will create sustainable results and a positive relationship with food just takes a little bit of time. Trial and error will come off the back of what in the past was seen as 'off plan', but for us we say #itsfine to adjusting, tweaking and changing things as often as you need. Our job is not only to show you the 'how', but actually show you the way . . .

Let's use the example of learning how to drive. You first need to understand how a car moves forwards and backwards, then how you drive it safely and responsibly. However, the way you actually drive a car today is very different from how you did it at the start. We doubt you still hold the steering wheel at the ten to two position do you? You'll probably be passing or crossing your hands over the top of it like most of us do.

We are going to give you the skills and tools you need to see how it's possible to get from A to B, just like a driving instructor would do. When you know all that and you pass, how you then navigate yourself to that destination is totally down to you.

Next up, really think carefully about your routine. Your job, when you wake up, go to sleep, exercise, how much free time you have as well as what you enjoy and what you don't. Now think again, but this time consider what you have been taught by others that you have added to your routine, because we still suspect there's an element of you falling into old habits set out by your previous fad diet. It's actually a lot harder than you think because, for the first time in a long time, you're taking some reflective 'me' time. It can be really eye-opening.

The key things we want you to really consider at this stage are time and appetite. Those are two important parts of your life that in the past haven't been addressed or supported properly.

When it comes to time, how much of it (we don't mean free time) could you comfortably allocate to preparing your meals? Let's not forget that being where you are now is most likely having a huge, negative impact on you and your family's life. So we suggest trying to prioritise a decent amount of it to cooking. Pretty much everything can be frozen and, when thawed correctly, tastes just as good as if cooked fresh. Therefore, if you're able to, take a few hours at the weekend to get ahead of the game and batch prep. We know from the feedback we get that it's a great way of doing it. If your weekends are busy, you could plan in some prep each evening, which could consist of chopping and portioning out ingredients to later combine and cook. It can even be as easy as making your meal for the evening, but making a double or a triple portion, so you can keep those other servings in the fridge for the next few days.

Your appetite needs to be addressed from the get-go. This is the biggest change and tweak we see happening during the first month, as you start listening to your hunger. Very often you will realise that eating at 'X' time doesn't suit you. We've known people swear and live by the rule of breakfast, then a couple of weeks later realise they've only been eating it because they thought they needed to. For them and their morning routine and hunger, a coffee was all they needed. Hunger for them kicked in at lunchtime where they had a large calorie-rich meal, with dinner being the same, followed by an evening snack watching TV. We have also seen avid snackers realise that it was more out of habit and living a restrictive lifestyle that made them crave those sweet snacks. They then introduced more sweet-flavoured foods into their week and snacks were left in the past.

Once you have an idea about when you will be eating food, you can then start adding our recipes into your planner and building something that is a much more appropriate starting point.

the recipes

When it comes to our recipes, two things are going to happen to you. Your mouth is going to water and you're going to be in disbelief!

Once you start browsing through the whole range of recipes, you'll start to realise they contain a lot of the things you were told you couldn't have in the past. Things like sugar, for example, or substantial amounts of carbohydrates, as well as perhaps a combination of ingredients that for decades of your life have always been off limits, until now. But #itsfine because our recipes have been designed not to magically enhance physical weight loss, but to re-introduce you to things you really enjoy. To take you out of your fad diet comfort zone into a new reality where food is consumed for enjoyment and pleasure and not just for function.

Unlike every other fat loss recipe book you have bought or meal plan you have tried and failed on, we don't pretend that the ingredients in a recipe will contribute to your body burning fat in a better or worse way. Yes, we have provided you with recipes that include nutrient-dense ingredients, which ensure you're consuming foods that are nourishing for your body, but also meals that nourish your mind. The key is balance and to ensure you eat a wide range of meals and ingredients rather than just sticking to one or two favourites.

But the only way you'll be truly convinced that you can enjoy the foods you love guilt-free is to eat them, all the while experiencing results you never thought were possible. That way you'll get the validation you need to move forward saying #itsfine.

We have also taken many of your takeaway favourites, removed all the processed elements and re-created them using healthier ingredients. No, we haven't done this because you're never allowed to have a takeaway or a meal out, we've done it so that when you do eat things like burgers, curries, pizzas, creamy cheesy pastas or chocolate, you just feel normal. You see, whatever we are told we can't have or is restricted, we will crave, then when we crack and start eating it, we get those feelings of Last Supper Syndrome (see page 32) which lead to a weekend-long binge.

By normalising these types of meals and simultaneously achieving results while eating them, it will turn social events and being impulsive into something pleasurable and enjoyable, rather than stressful and problematic.

We also want you to fully embrace the fact that you cannot go off plan with our recipes. Treat them as a guideline, not as a strict list of ingredients that if not stuck to 100 per cent will prevent you from losing body fat. If on occasions you see a recipe that contains beef, but in your fridge you only have chicken, then #itsfine, have the chicken instead. If one of our curries catches your eye, but you don't like the oil used, then #itsfine, swap it for butter. There will be some of you that have allergies and intolerances, so it's important that you know you can adjust things around them. Whether that's using dairy-free/gluten-free options instead, or removing or interchanging sesame seeds or nuts, #itsfine.

We're always going to recommend that you follow our recipe as it's written, because it has been designed to not only taste great but also to be a good balance of ingredients. However, it's really not a deal-breaker and will not prevent you from being successful if you tweak it slightly.

Our recipes have been created in a range of servings, some individual, some many more. There are many reasons behind why we do this. You will get the benefit of it being less wasteful and more budget-friendly, as you can save money buying in bulk, but also because they are designed to be family-friendly and easier to prepare and cook. There is, however, a much more important reason behind it, which is moving you away from obsessive portion control. We've seen this happen a lot, and it may be something you have done yourself. You decide on a recipe, then you make yours separately, despite your family having the same thing, because you need to get the exact grams and calories perfect. That's using calories in a way we don't want. Instead, you'll cook it in a batch that equates to say four portions, then you will serve yourself a quarter of it using only your eyes. The chances of your portion not being exactly a quarter are high, but the amount you'll be out by won't be, and within any one week will still be within your range, so don't give it a second thought.

saying #itsfine to anything else

That's right, anything goes, and this is all, again, part of what works for you. Some people really like the concept of routine and making their week 100 per cent about our recipes. This isn't right or wrong and it's certainly not 'on plan' perfection. It's just something that works well for them and is their plan. There are no brownie points for doing this, your accountability is not the food but the weekly calorie range. We find that people who do this will always at some point start bringing in new foods. It's just that they needed to feel a bit more comfortable before they were ready to do something that still felt like going 'off plan'.

We love our recipes and we know you will, too, but if there is something you really enjoy outside of them, it's important to eat it. That could be a recipe you've seen online, or from another cookbook, it may even be food from a meal delivery company or from the supermarket. You may decide to enjoy it once or twice a week, or every day, it's really up to you. As long as you're aware of the calories it contains, you can just add that into your planner. This doesn't have to be planned either, it could be totally spontaneous, no guilt, no worries, no self-sabotage, #itsfine!

At first, this can take some getting used to. After all, it couldn't be further away from what you are used to. So, if need be, take your time, don't push it. If you start to feel a little uncomfortable, just take a step back and focus more on our recipes. Stay in your comfort zone but be mindful of the freedom you have to test the water with that piece of chocolate or tea and biscuits. Each time you say #itsfine, you will feel empowered and proud of yourself that you no longer conform to fad diet culture, and with every bite you take comes an inner strength that pushes you further and further away from that old way of thinking.

banking calories

Do you remember Laura from Chapter Five? The lady at work who looks great, never puts on weight and can eat what she wants? Part of what she did subconsciously is what we call 'banking calories'. This is essentially when you have some days that have fewer calories in them, either planned or as a by-product of you being less hungry or busier, which results in having some calories in reserve, banked in the pot. These are the hidden subconscious habits that Laura isn't aware of that you can really benefit from to help move away from fad diet culture.

This certainly is not us saying: 'Starve yourself all week and earn a pizza at the weekend.' Not at all. What banking calories does is offer perspective and helps you practically understand that all those times you'd quit or self-sabotaged in the past, you were actually still more than likely within your weekly calorie range and therefore in a calorie deficit.

For some of you, you'll plan your meals and end up at the lower end of your calorie range or even under it, just because of your appetite and how you eat. For others, you will be somewhere closer to the middle, but, in both cases, there are still calories left in the bank so to speak.

Let's say, for example, you fancy having your friends round for a takeaway at the weekend. It's the start of your week, so what can you do? Well, first off, you can just say #itsfine and enjoy the meal without changing anything in your week. You'll wake up the following day, think nothing of it and move forward with your life. If you aren't the sort of person that does this very often, then this won't prevent you from achieving your goals. But, if you're like Laura, who enjoys a takeaway every weekend, then there is a method to factoring this in and still being within your range, as long as you're being sensible. That's the key word here, sensible. Not an eating challenge and not a large pizza with two sides, huge pots of dips, two bottles of wine and a large tub of ice cream. Unless you're Dwayne Johnson your body isn't going to use that all up as energy!

Very simple changes to your week can accommodate this and show you, through the numbers, no damage is being done. For example, being more active. Something as simple as going for an evening stroll Monday to Friday for thirty-five minutes can equate to as many as 1,500 calories in the bank. Or, if you snack, then removing those items or reducing them can easily get to a similar number. Some people skip breakfast a few times a week and have more of a mid-morning snack or nothing at all until lunchtime. There is no end to how you can do it, so as long as it suits your lifestyle and doesn't cause a huge lapse in energy levels, fitness or concentration and doesn't affect your sleep, then we say #itsfine.

This really is the same as saving the money you earn each week. You could get paid and spend it evenly across the week Monday to Friday, or you could stay in all week watching the TV and have a very sociable weekend instead. The result is always going to be the same – you spend your money how you like, the same way as you eat food the way you enjoy.

recording and taking your stats

First things first, don't forgot all your NSVs (Non-scale Victories) as these are very important and should be at the forefront of your mind, day in, day out, during your journey. There's no getting away from it though, you want to lose body fat and we get that. It's going to happen, we just want you to use the number on the scales among a whole plethora of other variables to determine how well you're doing.

Undies at the ready and get taking those pictures – front, side and back. You'll hate doing this; we did as well. However, the one thing in common for everyone who doesn't do this is that they wished they had. Let us ask you something: 'Would you rather look and feel good or just weigh less?' Exactly . . . and fat loss has a nasty way of not showing on the scales even when your weighing strategy is spot on.

Right then, on the subject of a weighing strategy, let's talk about the scales and making sure you aren't playing the weight loss lottery. Guess what the number one reason is for feeling guilty on a diet? What gave you enough reason to chuck it all in and give up so early on? What makes you throw in the towel months down the line despite making heaps of progress? Those bloody scales! Actually, we can't blame them, unfortunately, it just comes down to you and your weighing strategy.

You weren't born obsessed with the scales, you were taught that. Now it's time to learn something new. We warmed you up to this in Chapter Two, but now we can reveal that it's monthly weigh-ins from now on. 'What?!' we hear you cry! Yep, you heard it right. Here's some context for you . . .

Have you ever heard about someone claiming to be able to eat 1,000 calories or less per day and never lose weight? You may even have felt this yourself. The main reason behind it is due to impatience and standing on the scales too often, not metabolism. We've had thousands upon thousands of emails and conversations with people about this and, when we dig deeper into their history and the most recent weeks and months leading up to these conversations, it's clear. They haven't been consistently eating 1,000 calories at all. It was a cycle of daily weigh-ins showing a loss, a gain, a loss, a maintain, etc., etc. And many did this two or three times every day. It's usually when Friday comes along, after fifteen different readings on the scales and no real pattern or loss, that they believe there is something wrong with their bodies and embark on a huge blowout during the weekend. But the science is inescapable here. If you put anyone who isn't suffering from an untreated hormonal condition, like hypothyroidism, on 1,000 calories every single day for a month, the scales will always show an enormous drop in weight.

There are far too many variables at play with daily and weekly weigh-ins. Tracking your weight monthly instead means you miss out on all the random ups and downs. It's often at these points you overthink and question the process, and that's what we don't want.

Things to note when using the scales from day one:

1. Make sure you don't weigh in post-blowout! Unlike all restrictive fad diets, with our plan you won't need to panic and eat a week's worth of food in one day before you begin. You'll be eating all your favourites from the start, so don't feel like you need to cram it all in. We aren't about promoting a massive drop on the scales instantly, so we don't rely on using an incorrect and irrelevant starting weight just so you can feel like a fat-burning machine during the first few days. So, with that in mind, be sensible with your lead-up to starting your plan and eat as you would normally do.

2. Always weigh yourself first thing in the morning. For obvious reasons really, as weighing so close to mealtimes and after a drink is not going to be ideal.

3. Get your kit off before you weigh yourself. We want to keep your weigh-ins as consistent as possible and wearing different clothes and footwear can really throw it off each month.

4. Go to the loo. We aren't talking about a number two, unless you need to, but do empty your bladder.

5. *Don't weigh following a takeaway, because often you'll have consumed a load of carbs and salt and this can massively increase the amount of water your body has stored. We're not saying don't have a takeaway, of course, but if your monthly weigh-in day falls the day after having one, wait a couple of days so that all the water weight has gone and your body has returned to normal.*

Finally, get the tape measure out. Not a deal breaker here but another great marker of progress. It's possible during certain months to lose inches but maintain your weight if you regularly strength-train, as you may actually be losing fat and gaining muscle. This is very common with people who are new to the gym and are just getting into weight training. Also, make sure you measure as close to the same areas as possible.

So, use a variety of different things to determine how well you're doing and really note and celebrate the mental health wins you're making around food. Imagine going an entire month without feeling guilty about your food choices. How good would a week, let alone a month be, without some kind of self-sabotage? You really are much more than a number, so please, no cheeky weigh-ins.

Chapter 7

A LIFETIME OF FOOD FREEDOM!

the way you've always wanted to do it!

It's time to get excited, it's time to get planning and then it's time to get cooking, saying #itsfine!

What an achievement it is already for you, right? You're about to do something that a few weeks ago you would never have even contemplated was possible on a fat loss journey!

We have worked hard to get you to this point and, more importantly, you have worked even harder, breaking down your barriers and past beliefs to jump in to saying #itsfine.

It's time to properly introduce you to John, co-founder of #itsfine and the man behind our recipes. Like all the team at #itsfine, John has had his own struggles with weight and has used those experiences to create meals that will not only satisfy your taste buds, but also move you away from fad diets for good:

I want to show you that food doesn't have to be bland and boring when aiming for weight loss results. Eating in a restrictive way, where you have to say no to the foods you love, will never lead to a long-term sustainable relationship with food.

So, I looked at the meals we all love to eat – those popular restaurant options or the recipes that get our mouths watering during an advert or Instagram post. Then I made tweaks to remove the processed bits, to make them more nourishing and lower in calories – but without resorting to tiny portions.

One of the biggest issues with fad diets is restriction, which results in you missing out on some of the most amazing flavours and textures that so-called 'off plan' ingredients can give you. I want to introduce you to these ingredients using new combinations to show you how wide the world of food can be.

I hope you enjoy these as much as we all do at team #itsfine.

don't create a new obsession!

We have seen this happen with lots of people at the start, which is why it's important to bring it up early on. When it comes to weighing your ingredients (which yes, you must do) and portioning out your individual meals, it's not like building a house where millimetre accuracy is essential for the end result. In other words, if the recipe says 10g of butter and you scoop out 12g, or even 15g, don't freak out! Do you need to scrape off the excess to ensure your fat loss results aren't affected? Of course not, #itsfine. Taking this more relaxed approach to cooking is very important, not just for building a positive relationship towards food, but also to ensure you aren't in the kitchen all day trying to make the scales drop or increase by one or two grams with every ingredient you use. Just remember though, common sense and staying accountable to your own journey is important here, because going over the weight required with all ingredients for every meal is going to cause some issues. But don't sweat the small stuff because over the course of every week these little imperfections will always balance out.

The same goes for portioning out individual meals. Let's say you make our amazing Peach Melba Overnight Oats (see page 108), which makes four servings. Once prepared, you then want to break it down into four meals to store in the fridge. What do you do? Do you need to pull out the kitchen scales? Nope, not at all. Just lay out your four containers and evenly dish out the mix going by eye. Will you inevitably end up with four portions containing different amounts and therefore weighing more or less than each other? Well, yeah, but #itsfine! You will only ever be talking about small variations in the total calories per portion, irrelevant variations when looking at the bigger picture of your week. Even if one of those portions was 50 per cent more than the others (it won't be) you will still finish within your tailored range.

serving sizes

Our recipes vary in the number of servings, ranging from one all the way up to eight. This has been done to open up a wider range of possible meals for you, allowing you to create meals that you may not be able to do if trying to make one portion. Just try using a quarter of a raw egg and you'll see what we mean!

We also want to make this economical with a goal of minimising food waste. Being flexible in the number of portions made will allow you to buy larger packs of ingredients (very often cheaper per gram or millimetre than the smaller packs) and means those more specialised ingredients get used up, rather than finding a half-used bottle at the back of the fridge six months later!

That said, though, you can reduce or increase the number of servings you make, just ensure the maths for the ingredient quantities is right.

eating with friends and family

This is so important and plays a massive part in you being able to sustain things long term, bringing the whole household into living the #itsfine lifestyle with you.

As we have touched on before, and something you may have written down as one of your goals – fad dieting, friends and family don't mix. We have been there, sitting down to plain chicken, boiled rice and steamed broccoli, it's not too appealing to a ten-year-old or your best mate as part of dinner time!

This is where we are completely different, because making it family-friendly was one of our most important considerations when creating #itsfine. Not only will it be much easier to eat and socialise with these recipes, we are also confident your family and friends will be begging you to cook our meals!

You're not going to feel alone now with your food choices, because having that support from those near and dear to you, all of you enjoying the same meals together, will bring that sense of normality back into your journey and will help so much with getting you to your goals. That's why we'd like you to get the whole household involved as much as possible and eat together as often as you can. Just remember, back to portioning things out, don't spoil the moment by popping kitchen scales under each person's plate! Our advice, if you have made four servings, a quarter from the pan for you, then dish the remainder out to the family.

don't overthink it!

So that's it, you now have the tools you need to start enjoying delicious food, plus a library of amazing meals to get you going.

It's going to feel strange at the start, seeing ingredients you didn't think you could eat or meals you were previously told would stop your progress in its tracks. But you know better than that now, don't you? It's all calories, whatever you put into your body. When you realise that and stop over-analysing it, comparing a recipe to the 'rules' that fad diet culture has told you in the past, you really will be living the #itsfine lifestyle.

Food should be enjoyable and it should never feel like a chore to be on a weight loss journey. It should still mean new tastes, exciting new ingredients and new ways to prepare them. When you can have all that, all the while eating things you picked because you love to eat them, and still reach your targets, well that's the goal for all of us, isn't it?!

your weekly planner template

We don't just want you to plan, we want you to record – so we've created an example template for you to recreate each week. Treat this much more as a mini-diary that enables you to not only remain organised, but also recap on your progress to building a positive relationship with food.

The structure is totally down to you: just enter in your calorie range and then start mapping out the recipes you want in the first column for the day. We aren't telling you HOW or WHAT to eat, so you won't see a generic rule of thumb like your typical three, four or five meals and snacks per day – not with us! In the second column, embrace change and going with what's usually referred to as 'off plan' by listing what you said #itsfine to outside of our recipes. Keep a record of how you felt from what you ate that day and be honest, even if it seems negative. Looking back on this a few weeks down the line will let you know how far you've come and help you see food in a completely different way as you note it all down.

Once you get to the end of each day, tot up everything and detail the calories in the last column. You'll see as you go through the week just how different each day can be, and yet how easy it is to stay within your tailored weekly calorie range and make progress.

WEEK X	RECIPES	DID YOU SAY #ITSFINE?	HOW WAS TODAY?	CALORIES FOR THE DAY
MONDAY				
TUESDAY				
WEDNESDAY				
THURSDAY				
FRIDAY				
SATURDAY				
SUNDAY				
			WEEKLY CALORIE RANGE	
			WEEKLY CALORIE TOTAL	

some final words from us . . .

Now listen . . . just in case you still haven't realised . . . YOU are not the problem here. This pickle you've found yourself in, it isn't your fault. Not only that, despite what you think, being in this situation is much more normal than you think.

The reason nothing has worked for you is because, quite simply, it wasn't right for YOU. FOR YOU . . . Well, we believe 99 per cent of everything you have ever tried diet-wise isn't right for anyone, of course, but you know what we mean.

Whenever you feel is the right time for YOU to start saying #itsfine, please realise you've got us with you the whole time. This book is the voice of reason for you, it's a manual to use and reflect on any time you need it. In moments of uncertainty or doubt, go back through the pages to remind yourself of the facts, the past experiences you've forgotten, your goals and just how you got here in the first place. Old habits die hard and if you feel yourself slipping back into them (which you will), stop for a moment, take a breath, reread a chapter and reset.

Remember that if you plan for everything, then nothing can be off plan, right? Simply because you've already pre-empted and accepted it happening, so #itsfine.

The weight on the scales isn't your priority. Your mental health, your relationship with food, your family, friends, social life, career and a hundred other things are . . .

We could put a thousand of you in a room and, within the first month, all of you would have had different experiences and results, but #itsfine. Some will have committed 100 per cent to the process and breezed through. Some will have struggled to get going. Some will have lost their way slightly towards the end. BUT none of you will have done better or worse than others, because each one of your stories and journeys is incomparable. It's unique to YOU.

What's important now is that you don't feel alone, because you're not. You can engage with us through social media to share your experiences with the thousands of other people that are saying #itsfine.

This isn't a plan. This isn't a diet. This isn't a cookbook . . . this is a movement, a powerful moment in time, where you take back control of your life while disrupting the world of fad diets for good.

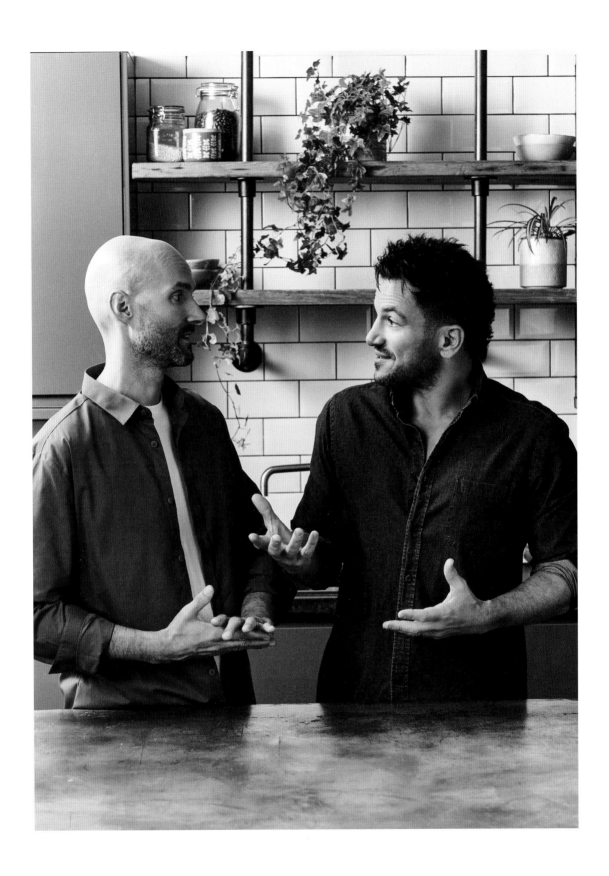

breakfast beauties

PB & J baked oats

Could breakfast get any better? That classic combination of peanut butter and jelly (that's jam for us Brits) but done the #itsfine way, turns this into a tasty way to start your day. Get your oats ready to bake the night before, then leave them in the fridge overnight for that perfect texture.

For the baked oats

50g porridge oats

1 tsp light soft brown sugar

250ml semi-skimmed milk

1 tbsp smooth peanut butter

For the jelly

75g ripe strawberries, diced

1 tsp runny honey

1 For the baked oats, place a saucepan over a low-medium heat and add the oats, sugar and milk. Stir well to combine, then cook the oats gently for around 10 minutes, stirring regularly. When they get lovely, creamy and thick, stir in the peanut butter, then you are ready.

2 Get a small baking dish and line it with nonstick baking paper. Pour in the oat mixture, smooth out into a nice even layer, then leave to cool for 30 minutes before chilling in the fridge overnight.

3 When you are ready to eat, preheat the oven to 150°C/130°C fan/ Gas Mark 2.

4 Transfer the baking dish to the oven and bake for 15 minutes or until golden brown.

5 Meanwhile, make the jelly. Simply add the strawberries and honey to a small saucepan and cook over a medium heat for around 5–8 minutes, stirring every now and then, until they get to that lovely sticky consistency.

6 Serve the warm strawberry jelly over the freshly baked oats.

shake my shakshuka with chorizo, roasted peppers and feta

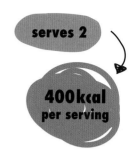

serves 2

400 kcal per serving

An absolute belter of a breakfast here and definitely not your average morning meal. Smoky and a little spicy, packed full of nutrients, it's a completely delicious way to start any day.

50g kale, roughly chopped

1 tbsp olive oil

½ white onion, finely diced

50g cooked chorizo ring, finely diced

1 garlic clove, finely chopped

1 tsp smoked paprika

½ tsp ground cumin

A pinch of chilli powder (or to taste)

70g roasted red pepper, diced

300g tinned chopped tomatoes

4 medium eggs

30g feta cheese

A small handful of coriander (leaves picked)

Salt and ground black pepper

1 Blanch the kale in a pan of lightly salted boiling water for a minute, then drain and leave to one side.

2 In a large frying pan, add the oil and then the onion and chorizo. Fry over a medium heat for 5 minutes before adding in the garlic and spices. Stir well to combine while frying for a further minute, then add the kale, red pepper and tomatoes. Season with a good pinch of salt and pepper and simmer for a few minutes. Break up any big chunks of tomato.

3 Make 4 wells in the sauce and crack the eggs into them, then cover the pan and leave to simmer for 5 minutes so that the eggs cook through to your liking.

4 Serve each portion with a crumble of feta and a scattering of coriander.

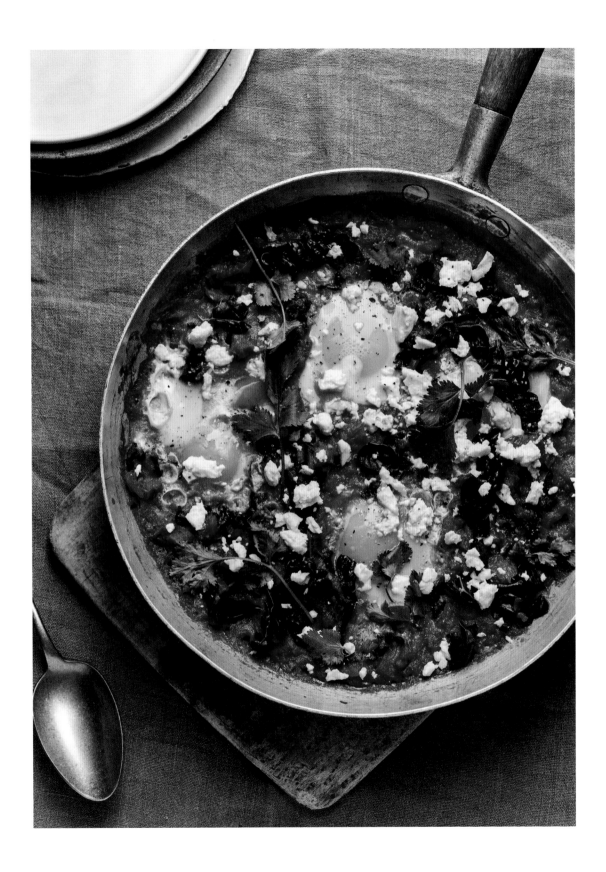

fine and fabulous french toast

serves 1

495kcal per serving

Who would have thought it? French toast on a diet! It's one of those dishes that's normally packed full of fat and calories, but our version is low in sugar and full of protein and fibre instead. And it's still a delicious treat any day of the week.

1 medium egg

80ml unsweetened almond milk

½ tsp ground cinnamon

25g protein powder

1 tsp vanilla extract

2 medium slices of sourdough bread

10g unsalted butter

A large handful of fresh raspberries

2 tbsp natural yogurt

1 Crack the egg into a bowl along with the milk, cinnamon, protein powder and ½ teaspoon of the vanilla extract. Give that a good mix until smooth, then add it to a shallow tray. Lay in the sourdough slices and let them soak up all the liquid, turning them over and leaving for 5 minutes to get the maximum effect.

2 Place a large frying pan over a medium heat and, when hot, add in the butter and let it melt. Carefully lay in the soaked bread and fry for 2-3 minutes on each side, until lovely and golden.

3 Transfer the cooked French toast to a plate and top with the fresh raspberries. Mix the yogurt with the remaining ½ teaspoon of vanilla extract and drizzle over the top. Tuck in!

Top Tip: Don't fancy the protein powder? That's never a problem, you can just leave it out and the calories will drop to 380kcal per serving.

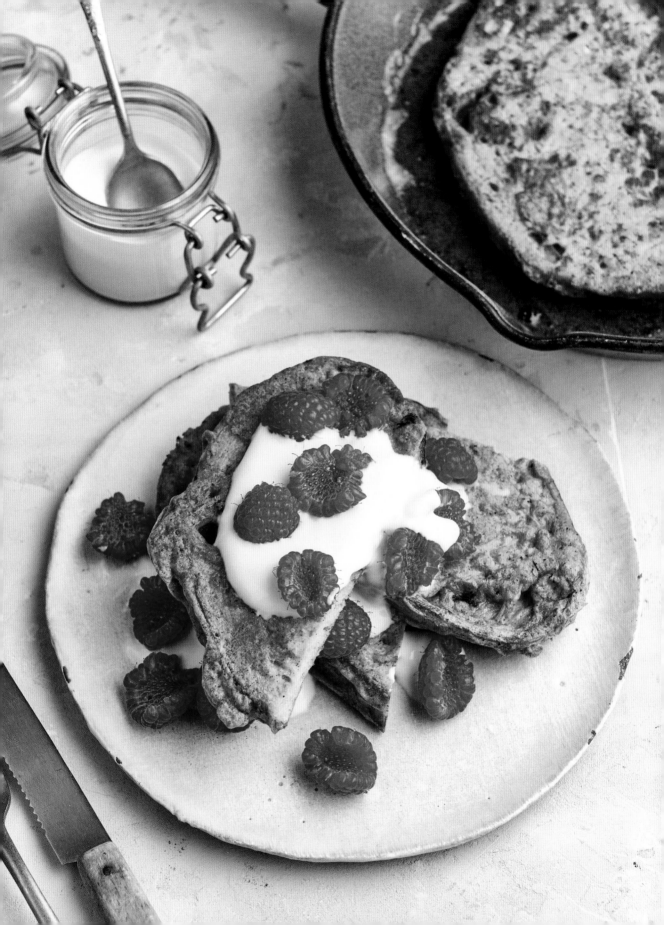

the McDaddy muffin

The ultimate breakfast (in our opinion at least). The homemade hash browns make this one a real treat and are a delicious addition to any morning feast – and all without a golden arch in sight!

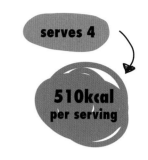

serves 4

510kcal per serving

For the hash browns
350g white potatoes
1 tbsp plain flour
1 tbsp olive oil
Salt and ground
  black pepper

For the pork patties
320g minced pork
  (5 per cent fat)
2 tsp dried sage
1 tbsp olive oil
4 Cheddar cheese slices

To finish and serve
4 medium eggs
1 tbsp olive oil
4 muffins, split in half

1 For the hash browns, peel the potatoes, then coarsely grate them. Place in a clean tea towel and squeeze out the excess liquid by twisting the tea towel. Place the grated potato in a bowl and season well with salt and pepper, then stir in the flour until combined.

2 Add the oil to a large frying pan. Place a cookie cutter the size of the muffins into the pan and pack it with a quarter of the potato mix, pressing it down well, then remove the cookie cutter. Repeat with the remaining potato mix to make 4 equal-size rounds, spacing them out in the pan. Fry gently for 3–4 minutes on each side or until they are golden brown and crisp.

3 Transfer the hash browns to a baking tray and keep warm in a low oven. Wipe out the frying pan with kitchen paper.

4 For the pork patties, add the minced pork to a bowl along with the sage and a good pinch of salt and pepper. Give it a good mix to combine, then divide and shape into 4 equal-size balls and press out into patties (about the same size as the muffins).

5 Add the oil to the frying pan you used for the hash browns and fry the patties for 4–5 minutes on each side, until cooked through. Top with the Cheddar cheese slices, then pop in the oven alongside the hash browns.

6 To finish, it's just a case of quickly frying the eggs in the oil and toasting the muffins. When everything is ready, pile it all into the muffins and serve. We would suggest a knife and fork for this one!

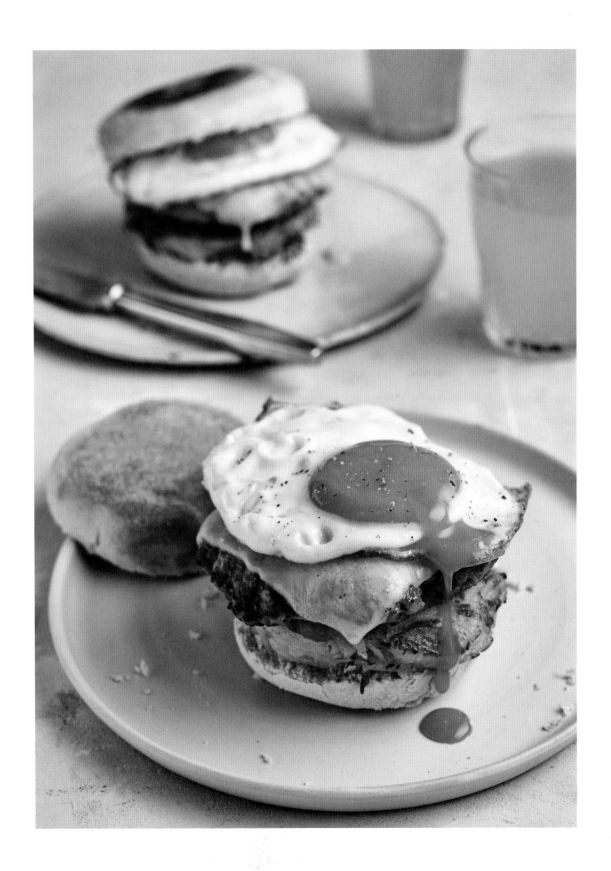

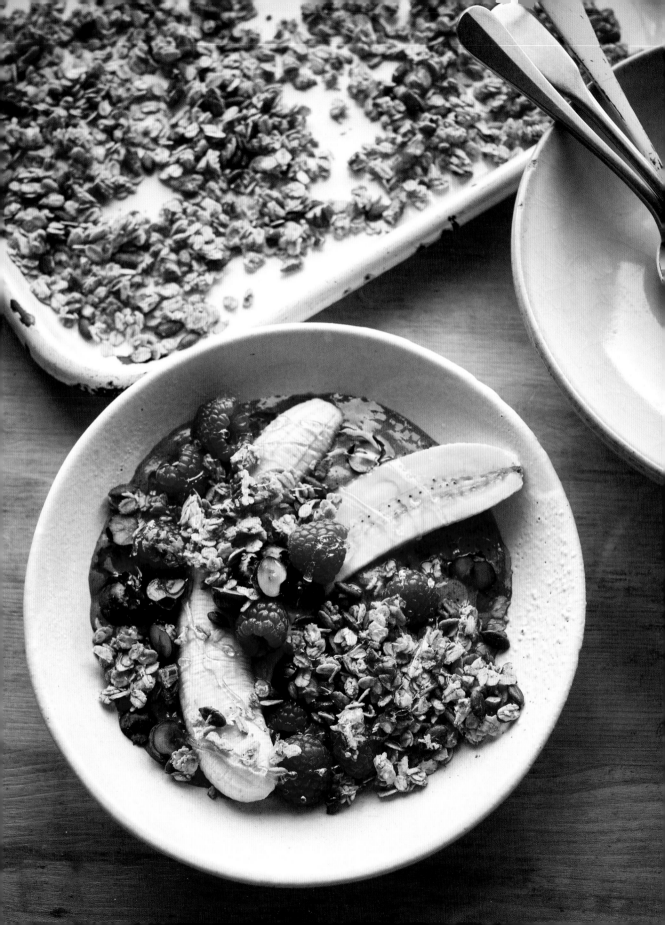

sundae brunch

An ice cream sundae for breakfast? That's the kind of healthy eating plan we want to follow! And this one isn't just delicious, it's also packed full of nutrients and fibre, so it's a massive win.

For the granola (makes approximately 180g - enough for 9 servings)

60g porridge oats

15g pumpkin seeds

15g chopped pecans

10g desiccated coconut

½ tsp ground mixed spice

Grated zest and juice of ½ orange

½ tbsp olive oil

20g runny honey

For the brunch

300g Greek yogurt

300g frozen berry smoothie mix

3 bananas

A handful of mixed fresh berries

60g granola (see above)

3 tsp runny honey

1 Preheat the oven to 150°C/130°C fan/Gas Mark 2. Line a baking tray with greaseproof paper.

2 Make the granola. Add the oats, pumpkin seeds, pecans, coconut, mixed spice and orange zest to a bowl and give it a mix. Add the orange juice, oil and honey and continue to mix, so everything gets really well combined.

3 Transfer the mix to a baking tray, spreading it out evenly, then pop it in the oven for 10-15 minutes. If it isn't quite golden and dry, pop it back in and bake for another 5 minutes.

4 Remove from the oven, leave to cool and then break it up. The granola will keep in an airtight container for at least a week.

5 To prepare the brunch, pop the yogurt and frozen berries into a blender or food processor and set it off. Let that whizz away until you get a lovely smooth mixture, then turn it off.

6 Add a couple of tablespoons of the berry yogurt mix into each serving bowl, then slice the bananas lengthways and place either side of the yogurt. Divide the rest of the yogurt between all 3 bowls, then top with the fresh berries. Share out the granola across each portion and finally drizzle over the honey.

peach melba overnight oats

If you love opening your fridge first thing in the morning and seeing your breakfast waiting there, then this is the recipe for you! It's even better when you know it tastes amazing and is also packed full of fibre, setting you up perfectly for the day ahead.

200g porridge oats

1 x 400g tin peach slices in juice, drained, with juice reserved

1½ tbsp maple syrup

400ml whole milk

200g natural yogurt

100g fresh raspberries

2 tsp desiccated coconut

A few basil leaves, thinly sliced

1 Share out the oats across 4 airtight containers, then split the peach juice, maple syrup, 300ml of the milk and all the yogurt out equally as well. Give each container a good mix, then cover and leave in the fridge overnight.

2 When you are ready to eat, add 25ml of the remaining milk into each container and mix to loosen up the oats.

3 Roughly chop half of the peaches and half of the raspberries and stir some through each portion of the oats, before topping with the remaining whole fruit pieces, the coconut and basil.

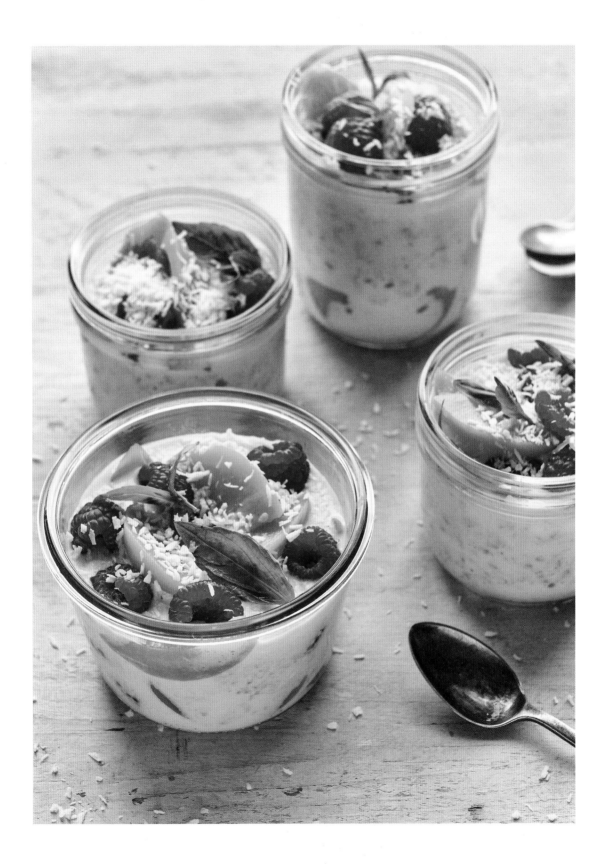

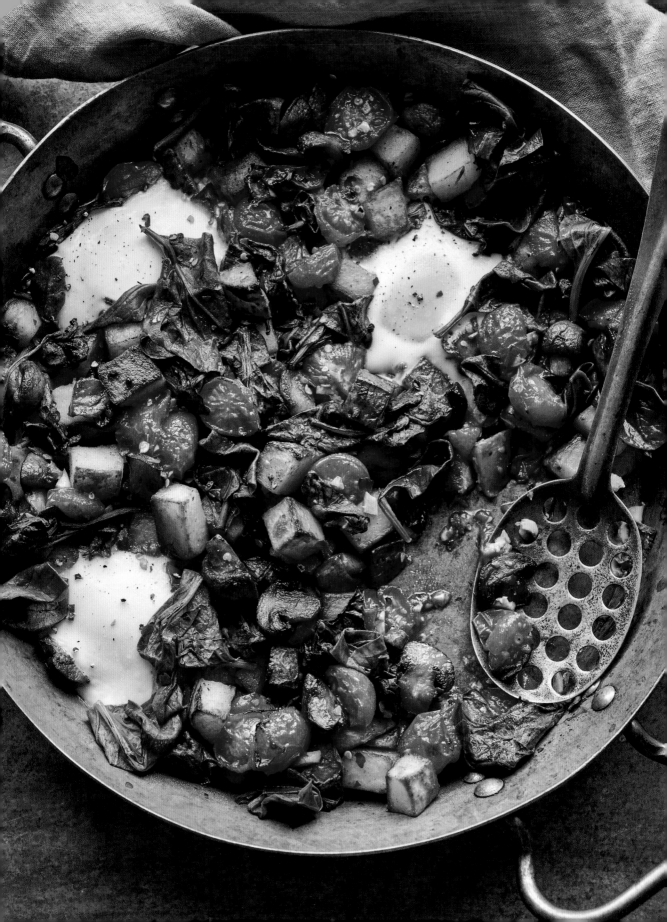

veggie breakfast bake

This is our kind of way to start the day! The combination of spuds, tomatoes and eggs is a real winner and will fill you up ready for the day ahead.

400g white potatoes, diced into 1cm chunks (no need to peel)

4 tsp olive oil

200g button mushrooms, halved

2 garlic cloves, finely chopped

A good pinch of dried chilli flakes, plus (optional) extra to serve

200g spinach (baby leaves)

200g cherry tomatoes, halved

4 large eggs

Salt and ground black pepper

1 Pop the potatoes into a pan of boiling water and cook for 5-8 minutes, until tender, then drain.

2 Place a large frying pan over a medium heat and, when hot, add the olive oil. Add the potatoes with a pinch of salt and pepper so you can crisp them up. After a few minutes, add the mushrooms, garlic and chilli flakes and give it all a good mix, then pile on the spinach to allow it to wilt.

3 Meanwhile, preheat the grill to high.

4 Once the spinach has wilted, add the tomatoes and continue to fry for a further couple of minutes before cracking the eggs straight into the pan – make 4 wells in the other ingredients and drop them in.

5 Pop the pan straight under the hot grill and let that cook away for 2-3 minutes, until the eggs are cooked to your liking. Add a few extra chilli flakes if you like it spicy, and dig in.

ben's banging breakfast tacos

Sometimes breakfast can be something completely different to the norm, and that's just what makes these tacos Ben's go-to choice.

For the refried beans

2 tsp olive oil

50g red onion, finely diced

1 garlic clove, minced

¼ tsp chilli powder (or to taste)

A pinch of ground cumin

1 x 400g tin haricot beans, drained and rinsed (around 235g drained weight)

A good pinch of salt

Juice of ½ lime

A large handful of chopped coriander leaves, plus extra to serve

For the pico de gallo

100g red onion, finely diced

1 jalapeño chilli, deseeded and finely diced

A pinch of salt

Juice of 1 lime

100g ripe tomatoes, finely diced

A good handful of chopped coriander

For the tacos

70g cooked chorizo ring, finely diced

8 small corn tortillas

1 large ripe avocado, peeled, stoned and sliced

1 To make the refried beans, add the oil to a saucepan over a medium heat, then add the onion and fry gently for around 5 minutes until softening. Add the garlic and spices and stir well, letting them fry out for about a minute, before adding in the beans and 2-3 tablespoons of water. Leave to simmer, covered, for about 10 minutes.

2 Next, take a fork and start to mash the beans up, so the whole mix gets lovely and thick. You want to be able to spoon it on to the tacos and spread it, like hummus. If it's a little too thick, add a splash more water; if it's too runny, just let it cook out for a little longer. When it's perfect, remove from the heat, add the salt and a squeeze of lime juice along with some chopped coriander, then leave to one side.

3 The pico de gallo is super simple. Just add the diced onion and chilli to a bowl along with the salt, then squeeze in the lime juice. Give it a good mix and let that sit for about 5 minutes, before stirring through the tomatoes and coriander.

4 The final bit of prep is the chorizo, so add it to a small cold pan and fry over a medium heat for around 5 minutes, until the oils are released and the chorizo is crispy.

5 Separate the tortillas, then restack and warm in a microwave on High for about 30 seconds. When they're ready, serve up each tortilla with a generous spoonful of refried beans and the same of pico de gallo. Add some slices of avocado and a few crispy chorizo bits to each along with a drizzle of the chorizo oil, then finish with a little more coriander. Tuck in and enjoy!

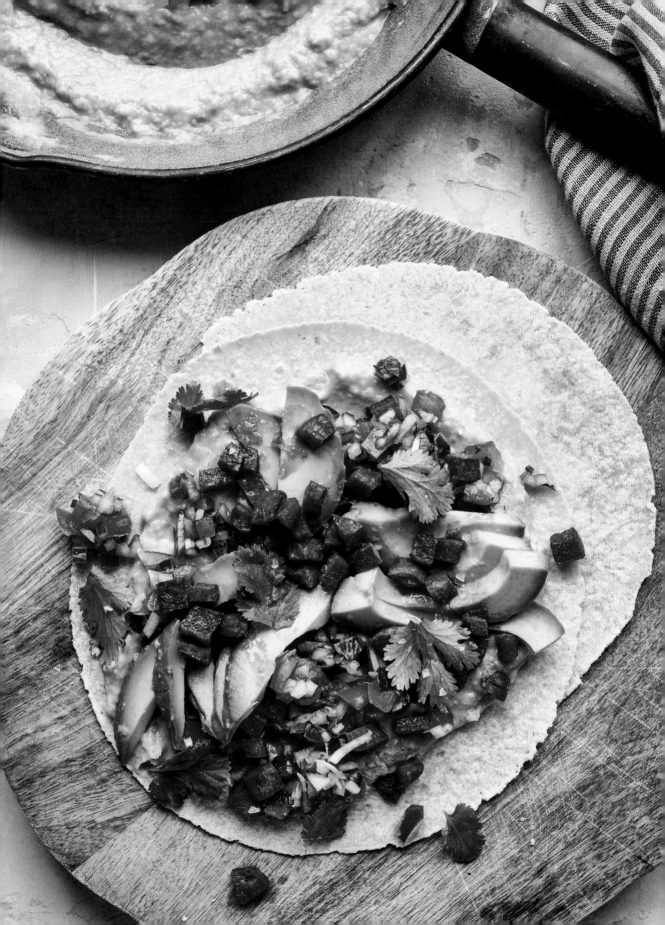

'no egg' pancakes with caramel bananas

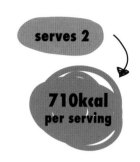

This vegan breakfast is a bit of us! We know #itsfine to eat, but also know that it shouldn't be every day. It's not as nutrient-dense as many of our others but can still be enjoyed on a weight loss journey.

For the pancakes

120g plain flour

1 tbsp baking powder

2 tbsp unsalted vegan butter, melted

240ml unsweetened almond milk

1 tbsp maple syrup

1 tbsp unsalted vegan butter

For the caramel

60g light soft brown sugar

2 tbsp unsalted vegan butter

40ml oat cream

1 banana, sliced, to serve

For smaller appetites, turn this into 3 servings at 475kcal per serving.

1 Get the pancake batter together first by adding the flour and baking powder to a large bowl. Give them a little whisk, then add in the melted butter, the almond milk and maple syrup. Make sure everything gets combined, then leave to one side for 5 minutes.

2 Meanwhile, for the caramel, place a heavy-based saucepan over a medium heat and add the sugar. As it melts, make sure you are continuously stirring with a wooden spoon as it will burn easily. When completely melted and light brown, add the butter. It will foam away but keep carefully stirring. When the butter has been incorporated, slowly and carefully add the oat cream while stirring. When all the cream is in, let it bubble away for another minute, then remove from the heat and leave to one side.

3 To cook the pancakes, place a nonstick frying pan over a medium heat. When hot, add half the butter and use half the batter to make 4 mini/small pancakes (keeping them separate in the pan). When they start to puff up and you see lots of bubbles coming through, that's the time to flip them, and they should be lovely and golden underneath. Cook for another couple of minutes on the other side, then remove them from the pan and repeat with the remaining butter and batter.

4 To serve, pile up the pancakes on 2 plates, top with slices of banana and then drizzle over that lovely caramel sauce.

Top Tip: You may find it easier to cook the pancakes individually or in pairs. If so, you can pop them in a warm oven once cooked to keep them hot, while you cook the rest. The pancakes will freeze perfectly once cooked and can be defrosted overnight, then reheated in the oven at 160°C/140°C fan/Gas Mark 3 for 10 minutes.

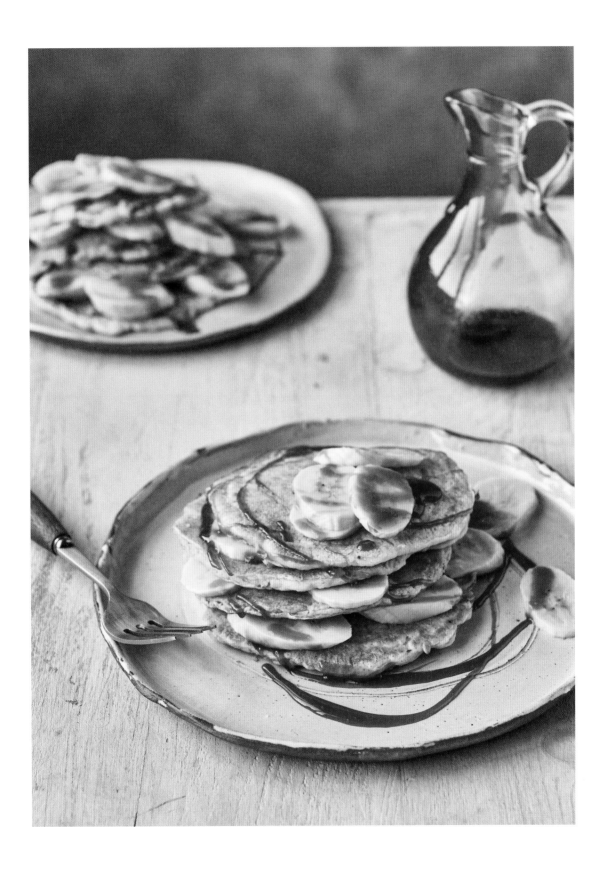

smoked salmon benny

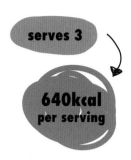

There is no getting away from it, this one will take a while to knock up and has a few tricky elements. But believe us, the end result is worth it. So take a Sunday morning, get the radio on and give this one a go.

For the potato pancakes
150g cold mashed potato
40g plain flour
½ tsp baking powder
70ml semi-skimmed milk
1 large egg
A small bunch of chives, finely chopped, plus a few extra to serve
1 tsp vegetable oil
10g unsalted butter
Salt and ground black pepper

For the hollandaise sauce
75g unsalted butter
1 large egg yolk
½ tsp white wine vinegar, plus an extra little splash for poaching the eggs
Juice of 1 lemon
A pinch of salt

To serve
6 medium eggs
180g thinly sliced smoked salmon

1 For the potato pancakes, pop the mashed potato, flour and baking powder in a large bowl. In a separate bowl, whisk together the milk and egg. Add the wet mix into the dry ingredients along with the chives, then mix well to combine into a thick-ish batter. Season with salt and pepper.

2 Place a large frying pan over a medium heat and add half of the oil and butter. When hot, spoon in 3 large dollops of the batter (using roughly half of the total amount), keeping them separate in the pan. Leave for 2–3 minutes before flipping – you want them to be lovely and golden brown and crisp. Cook the other side for the same time, then transfer to a plate and keep warm in a low oven. Add the remaining oil and butter to the pan and cook the other 3 pancakes in the same way.

3 While they stay warm in the oven, make the hollandaise sauce by gently melting the butter in a small saucepan, then remove from the heat. Place another pan filled with around 2.5cm of water on the hob and bring to a gentle simmer. Pop a heatproof bowl over the pan of water and add the egg yolk to the bowl. Using a whisk, start to beat the yolk, then add in the vinegar. Continue to whisk while you slowly trickle in the melted butter, taking your time over it and allowing the mixture to thicken. When all the butter is used up, add a squeeze of lemon juice just to loosen it a little, along with the pinch of salt.

4 Now it's just a case of getting the poached eggs done. So in a large pan of simmering water, add a little splash of white wine vinegar and give the water a good swirl. Carefully crack in the eggs (cook them in batches of 2 at a time), then leave to gently simmer for around 3 minutes, until the white has set. If serving all

For smaller appetites, turn this into 6 servings at 320kcal per serving.

the portions at the same time, remove the cooked eggs 30 seconds early and leave in a bowl of iced water while you cook the rest. Refresh them back in the simmering water for 30 seconds before serving.

5 To serve, place 2 pancakes on each plate, top each one with a portion of smoked salmon and a poached egg, and then pour over some of the hollandaise sauce. Finish with a few more chopped chives.

Top Tip: The pancakes will freeze perfectly once cooked and can be defrosted overnight and then reheated in the oven at 160°C/140°C fan/Gas Mark 3 for 10 minutes.

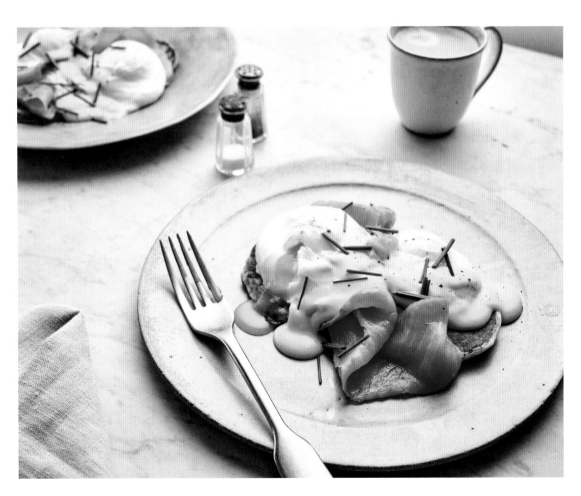

sunshine smoothie bowl

This bowl of deliciousness is not just full of fresh fruit, but is also jam-packed with fibre and nutrients.

2 frozen bananas
(see Top Tip)
200g frozen mango
chunks
150ml light coconut milk
30g flaxseeds
100g fresh blueberries
130g fresh pineapple
pieces
2 tsp chia seeds
1 tsp desiccated coconut

1 This really is so simple to prepare. Add the frozen bananas and mango chunks, the coconut milk and flaxseeds into a blender and set that off. Let it whizz away until everything is combined and you have a lovely smooth mixture. Share that out between 2 bowls.

2 Now you can just top the smoothie bowls with all the other ingredients, dividing them equally between each portion. Make each bowl as bright and beautiful as you feel!

Top Tip: When you freeze the bananas, make sure they're peeled and chopped up into chunks beforehand.

baked granola bars

These baked granola bars are the perfect go-to breakfast. They will keep in an airtight container for 3–4 days, so are great to make in advance.

150g pitted dates,
roughly torn
1 tsp ground cinnamon
½ banana
50g dried cranberries
50g pumpkin seeds
85g ground flaxseeds
30g cacao nibs
15g chia seeds
20g toasted rice cereal
70g porridge oats

1 Preheat the oven to 170°C/150°C fan/Gas Mark 3½ and line a square baking tin (about 20 x 20cm) with greaseproof paper.

2 Pop the dates into a small saucepan with the cinnamon and 200ml of water. Bring to the boil, then simmer for 5 minutes, before removing from the heat and mashing.

3 Add the banana to a bowl and mash. Add all the other ingredients along with the mashed dates, then mix well to combine.

4 Spoon the mixture into the lined baking tin and spread evenly. Bake for 20 minutes until golden brown.

5 Remove from the oven and leave to cool slightly before taking out of the tin and cutting into portions to serve.

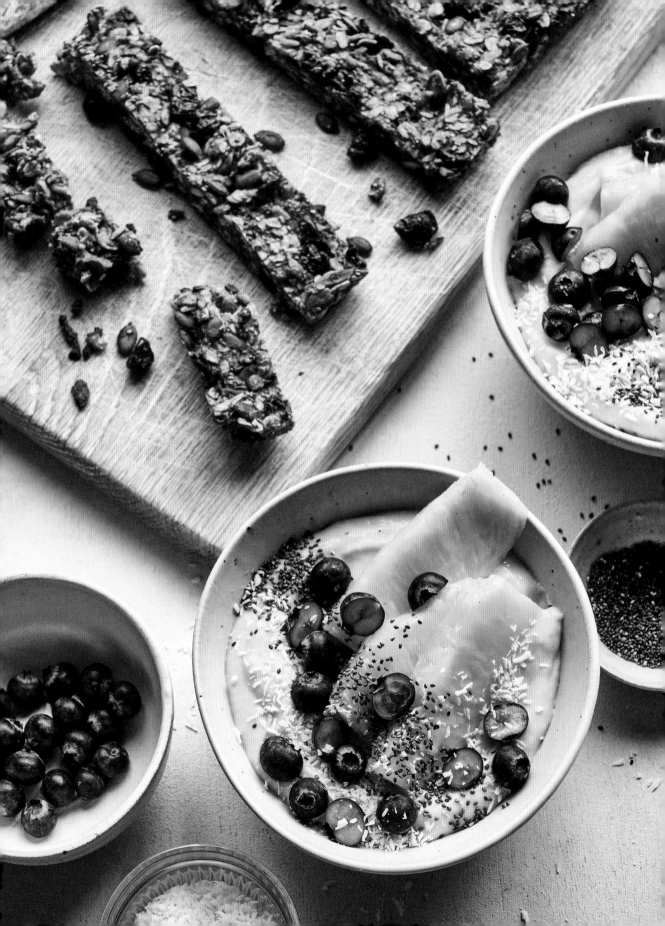

lunches to lose with

the ultimate toasted cheese sandwich

serves 1

600kcal per serving

OK, so we know by now that food, in the main, should be nutrient-dense. However, we also know that food should be delicious, and it's all about finding the right balance that leads to sustainability. So, we call this a special occasion sandwich to enjoy every now and then rather than all the time, and that's a balance we can deal with!

1 tbsp unsalted butter, softened

2 medium slices of sourdough bread

25g red onion and chilli jam (page 232)

30g Cheddar cheese, grated

20g Gruyère cheese, grated

10g Parmesan cheese, finely grated

For smaller appetites, split all the measurements in half, for example, using one slice of bread instead of two. This will get the calories down to 300kcal.

1 Set a large frying pan over a medium heat. Spread the butter over the outsides of the bread slices (the sides you will see at the end) to give them both a good coating. On the inside (un-buttered side) of one slice, add the jam and the Cheddar and Gruyère. Top with the other slice (buttered-side facing out) and carefully transfer to the pan.

2 Leave to cook on one side for 2-3 minutes, using a spatula or turner to press down every now and then. Carefully flip the sandwich over and repeat on the other side.

3 The final step is to remove the sandwich and add the Parmesan to the pan in a thin layer. Let that start to melt before laying the sandwich back on it. Give it another minute or so to really melt into the bread, then slide the turner underneath, making sure you get all that lovely crispy Parmesan off with it, and transfer to a plate.

4 Cut in half and dig in. Watch out for that hot melty cheese!

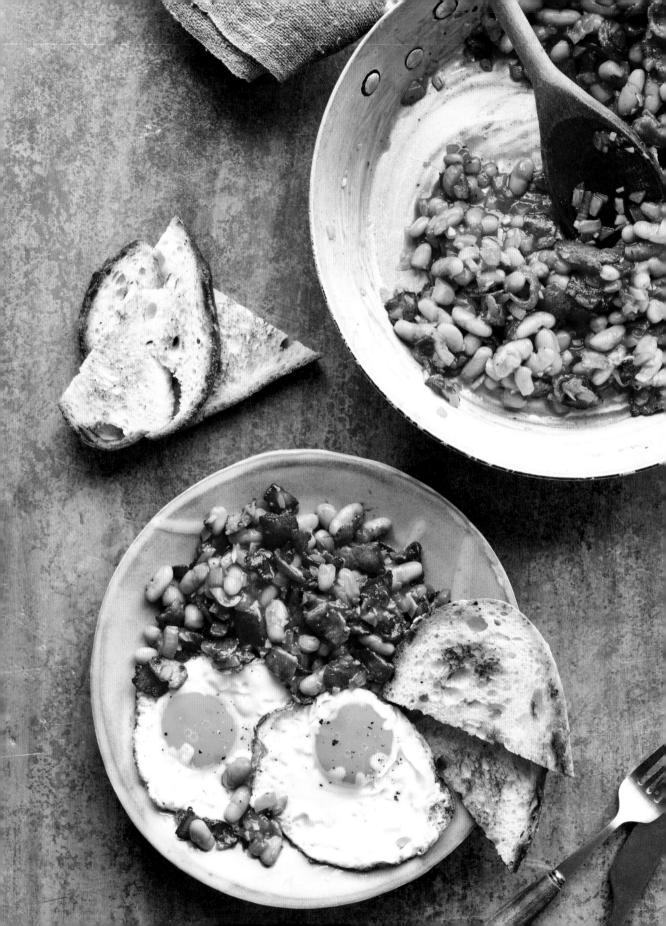

smoky beans with eggs

serves 3

500 kcal per serving

Trust me, these are nothing like the beans from a tin! Smoky and rich, they go so well with eggs and toast. This is a weekend winner if I have ever seen one. Perfect for batch prepping, the cooked beans will keep in the fridge for at least a week.

200g smoked streaky bacon rashers, diced

1 large white onion, diced

3 garlic cloves, diced

1 x 400g tin cannellini beans, drained and rinsed

1 tbsp light soft brown sugar

3 tbsp BBQ sauce

1 tbsp English mustard

1 tbsp unsalted butter

6 medium eggs

3 medium slices of sourdough bread

1 Heat a nonstick saucepan over a medium-high heat until hot, then start to fry the bacon for about 5 minutes, until it's nice and crispy. Now add the onion and garlic and continue frying for 2–3 minutes.

2 Add the cannellini beans to the pan along with the brown sugar, BBQ sauce and mustard. Give this a good mix, then add a little splash of water to make a sauce. Bring to the boil, then turn down to a simmer and allow it to tick away, while you turn your attention to the eggs.

3 In a nonstick frying pan, melt the butter over a low heat, then fry the eggs to your preference. When the eggs are nearly ready, whack the sourdough in the toaster.

4 Load up a large serving bowl (or individual bowls) with the beans, top with the eggs and serve with the toast.

new york deli in your belly bagel

serves 1

475kcal per serving

This is, in our opinion at least, the king of sandwiches! Such a delicious range of things piled into a bagel, topped off with a lovely zingy mustard mayo. Sauerkraut may be something you aren't too sure about, but if you haven't had it in one of these before, then you have got to give it a go.

1 plain white bagel
1 tbsp sauerkraut
4 slices of pastrami
2 tsp mayonnaise (page 231)
1 tsp Dijon mustard
25g Emmental cheese, thinly sliced
1 gherkin, drained and sliced

1 Carefully split the bagel and pop it in the toaster until it's lovely and golden brown.

2 When it's ready, cover the base with the sauerkraut and then add the pastrami. Combine the mayonnaise and mustard in a small bowl and cover the pastrami with it, then top with the Emmental and gherkin slices.

3 Pop the bagel lid on and take a bite.

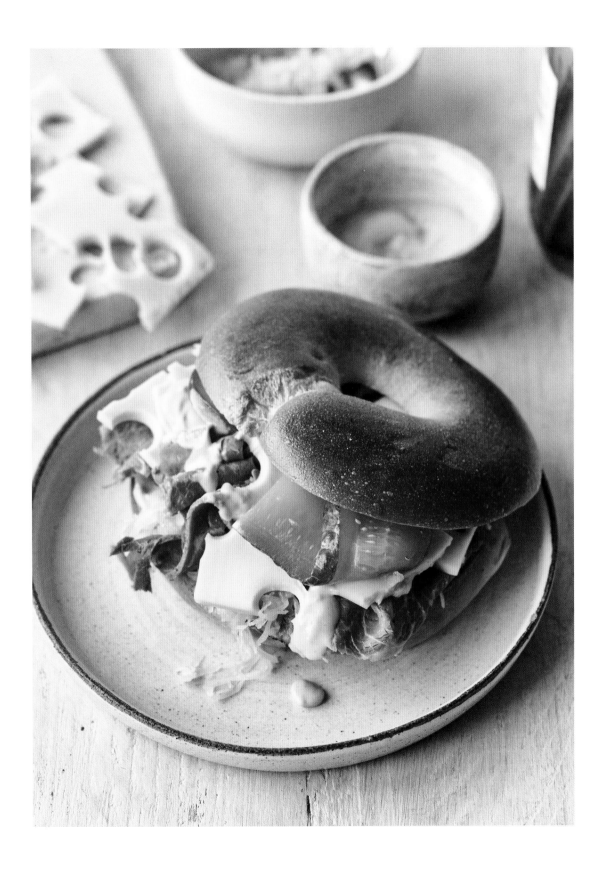

our perfect poke bowl

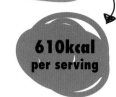

serves 2

610kcal
per serving

We know raw fish may not sound like your ideal ingredient, but when you leave it in the marinade wonderful things happen! Plus, the flavour is unreal.

For larger appetites (610kcal per serving)

140g basmati rice

220g skinless
   salmon fillet

Juice of 1 lime

1 tsp maple syrup

2 tsp light soy sauce

½ tsp white wine vinegar

70g carrot, grated

70g cabbage, grated

80g pickled courgettes
   (page 230)

120g kimchi (page 229)

80g edamame beans

2 tsp spicy mayo

For smaller appetites (450kcal per serving)

100g basmati rice

165g skinless
   salmon fillet

Juice of 1 lime

1 tsp maple syrup

2 tsp light soy sauce

½ tsp white wine vinegar

55g carrot, grated

55g cabbage, grated

60g pickled courgettes
   (page 230)

95g kimchi (page 229)

65g edamame
   beans (podded)

1 tsp spicy mayo

1 Cook the rice as per the packet instructions, then drain and leave to cool for 5-10 minutes.

2 While the rice cooks, dice the salmon into 1cm cubes and add to a bowl with the lime juice, maple syrup, soy sauce and vinegar. Stir to combine and leave to sit for 5 minutes.

3 When the rice is ready, load this up in one corner of each serving bowl, sharing it evenly, then add the other vegetable ingredients around the bowls.

4 Finish by adding the marinated salmon over the top (along with a drizzle of any leftover marinade), then add a small dollop of spicy mayo to each bowl and serve.

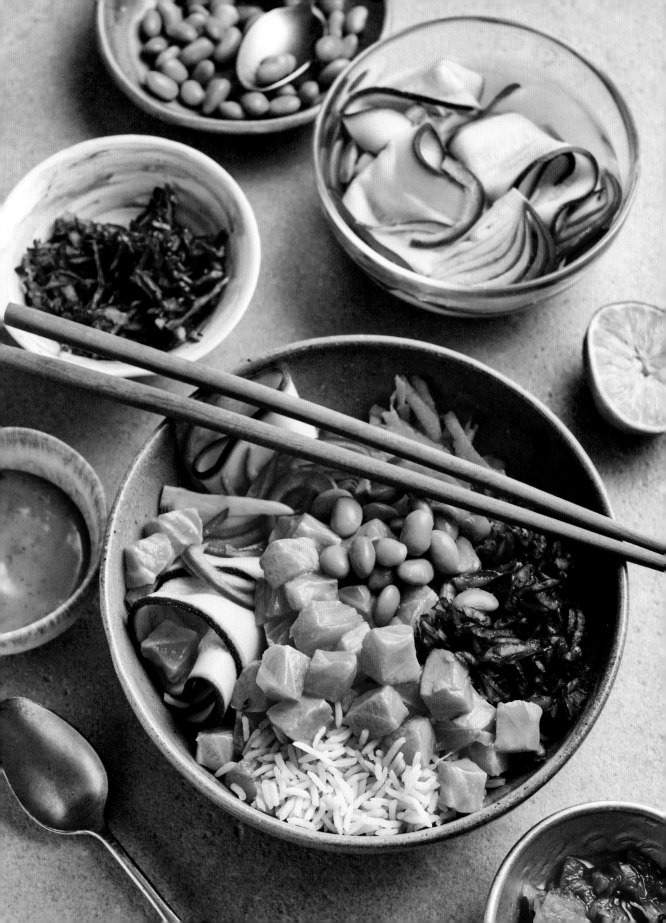

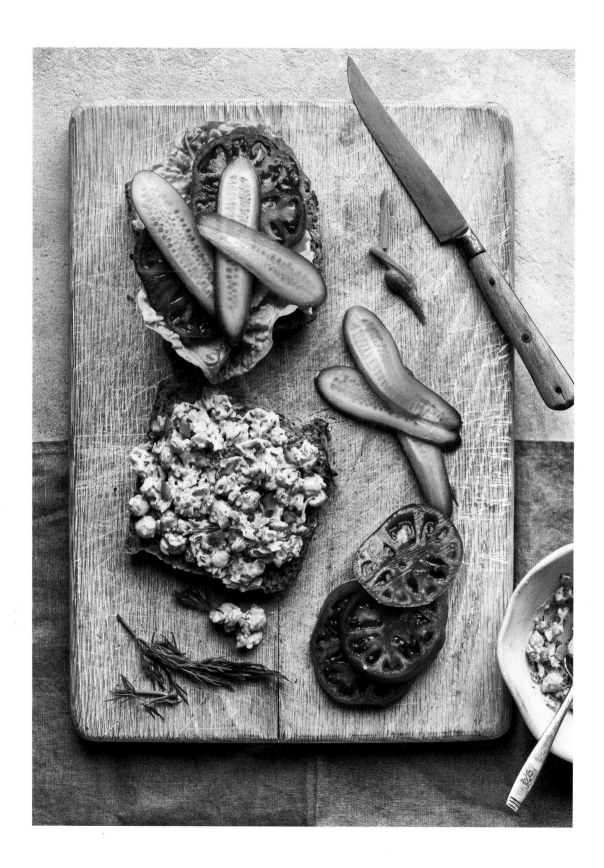

chickpea salad sandwich

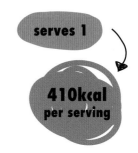

serves 1

410kcal per serving

This super simple lunch idea can be knocked up in a matter of minutes, it's 100 per cent vegan and is completely delicious.

80g (drained weight) tinned chickpeas, drained and rinsed

1 tbsp vegan mayonnaise

1 tsp Dijon mustard (make sure it's vegan-friendly!)

1–2 gherkins, drained and finely diced

A few thin slices of red onion

1 tsp chopped dill

2 slices of wholemeal bread

A few tomato slices

A few cucumber slices

½ baby gem lettuce, separated into leaves

Salt and ground black pepper

1 Add the chickpeas to a bowl and give them a good mash up with a potato masher or a fork. Don't worry if you leave a few whole chickpeas in there, you just want to get most of them squashed.

2 Add in the mayo, mustard, gherkins, red onion and dill. Give that all a good mix and season with a pinch of salt and pepper.

3 Now it's just a case of spooning the mix on to one of the slices of bread, covering with tomato and cucumber slices and the lettuce leaves, then topping off with the other slice of bread.

huevos rancheros

More importantly, this should be called 'leftovers huevos rancheros', as this one is perfect for all those bits and bobs you have left over in the fridge.

100g cooked chorizo ring, finely diced

4 spring onions, white and green parts separated, thinly sliced

2 handfuls of cherry tomatoes, quartered

A pinch or two of dried chilli flakes (to taste)

2 tsp olive oil

4 medium eggs

Ground black pepper

1 This couldn't be any simpler. Just add the chorizo to a large frying pan over a medium heat, leaving it to fry until you start to see the oil come out and it starts to go crispy.

2 Next, add in the white parts of the spring onions and the cherry tomatoes along with a pinch or two of chilli flakes, depending on how spicy you like it. Leave that to fry until the tomatoes start to break down, around 5 minutes.

3 To finish, place a separate large frying pan over a medium heat and, when hot, add the oil. Crack in the eggs and fry them to your liking.

4 Share the cooked chorizo and veggie mixture out between 2 plates and then top with the cooked eggs, a pinch of pepper and the green parts of the spring onions.

Top Tip: The great thing about this recipe is how completely versatile it can be. The vegetables can be anything you have to hand, and the calories from these are so low, you can go wild. Chuck in ½ deseeded, chopped red pepper (20kcal) or get some greens in there with a large handful of fresh spinach (10kcal).

You could even take this to the next level and turn it into a more substantial meal, with 100g of hot cooked long-grain rice (140kcal) mixed through.

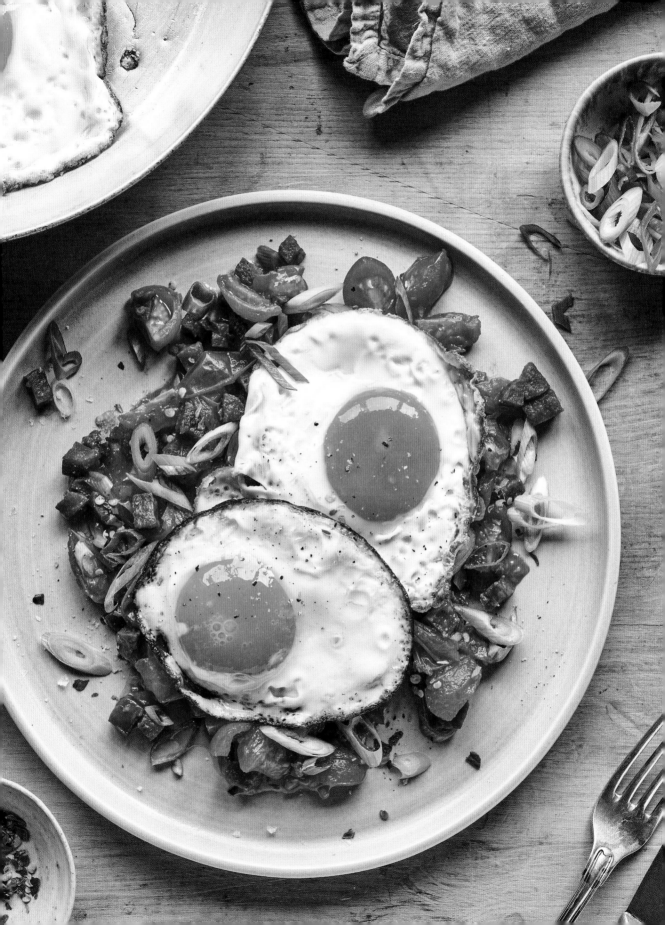

sweet and sticky chicken tenders sandwich

serves 2

700kcal per serving

This is packed full of flavour and will feel like a treat, but it shouldn't do. It's just a delicious chicken sandwich.

For larger appetites (700kcal per serving)

1 tbsp plain flour

1 tbsp Cajun seasoning

1 large egg

60g panko breadcrumbs

300g boneless, skinless chicken breasts

2 tsp olive oil

30g runny honey

1 tbsp hot sauce

2 white sub rolls

20g mayonnaise (page 231)

1 baby gem lettuce leaves

½ red onion, sliced

1 large vine tomato, sliced

For smaller appetites (495kcal per serving)

2 tsp plain flour

2 tsp Cajun seasoning

1 medium egg

40g panko breadcrumbs

200g boneless, skinless chicken breasts

1 tsp olive oil

15g runny honey

½ tbsp hot sauce

2 seeded burger buns

10g mayonnaise (page 231)

1 baby gem lettuce leaves

½ red onion, sliced

1 large vine tomato, sliced

1 Preheat the oven to 180°C/160°C fan/Gas Mark 4. Line a baking tray with greaseproof paper.

2 Get yourself 2 large plates and 1 large bowl. Add the flour and Cajun seasoning to one plate and mix to combine. Crack the egg into the bowl and whisk, then add the breadcrumbs to the remaining plate.

3 Cut the chicken breasts into strips around 1-2cm thick and add them to the flour plate. Make sure they all get a good coating, then move into the egg, again ensuring they are well covered. Allow the excess egg to drip off, then move them into the breadcrumbs. Carefully toss the chicken pieces in the crumbs, making sure you get a good coating all over. You can do this all in one go or do the full process one piece (or a few pieces) at a time, if you prefer.

4 Transfer the breaded chicken pieces to the lined baking tray before carefully drizzling over the olive oil. Pop them in the oven for 20 minutes, until golden and crisp.

5 When the chicken is ready, mix the honey and hot sauce together in a small bowl and then spoon over the cooked pieces. Now you can just pile it all into the sub rolls or burger buns, along with a dollop of mayonnaise, a few lettuce leaves and a few slices of red onion and tomato. Tuck in and enjoy!

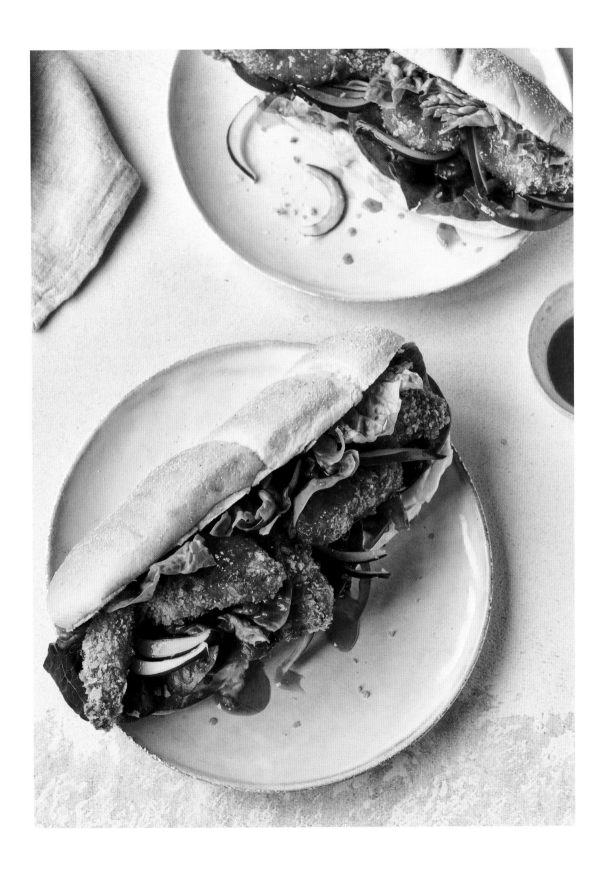

crispy tofu ramen

A Japanese ramen soup is a great way to get your veggies in and a brilliant dish to take with you on the go. Make sure you opt for a firm tofu that holds its shape when cooking.

280g firm tofu

500ml boiling water

1 vegetable stock cube

1 tsp miso paste

2 garlic cloves, cut in half

2.5cm piece of fresh root ginger, peeled and sliced

A small bunch of coriander, stalks and leaves separated

2 tbsp light soy sauce

2 tbsp vegetable oil

130g mushrooms, sliced

90g baby corn, roughly chopped

80g bean sprouts

150g straight-to-wok medium noodles

2 tsp cornflour

2 medium eggs

1 red chilli, sliced (and deseeded if preferred)

1 A couple of hours before you are going to cook this, cut the tofu into roughly 1cm cubes and place in a single layer within a clean folded tea towel. Place a board on top and then something heavy like a saucepan and leave to press out any excess water.

2 When you are ready to cook, start by making the broth. Add the boiling water to a saucepan along with the crumbled stock cube, the miso, garlic, ginger, coriander stalks and 1 tablespoon of the soy. Let that simmer for 10 minutes, then strain into another pan (discard the flavourings), leaving it to one side over a very low heat.

3 In a wok or large frying pan, add 1 tablespoon of the oil and, when hot, add the mushrooms, baby corn and bean sprouts. Stir-fry over a high heat for a few minutes, then pop the noodles in and continue to stir-fry until they have broken apart. Divide the veggies and noodles between 2 serving bowls and set aside.

4 Wipe out the pan with a piece of kitchen paper and add the remaining tablespoon of oil. Place the tofu cubes into a bowl, add the remaining soy sauce along with the cornflour and toss them well to coat. When the oil is hot, carefully add the tofu to the pan and stir-fry over a high heat for 8–10 minutes, turning regularly, until lovely, golden and crispy.

5 While the tofu cooks, pop the eggs into a small pan of boiling water and cook for around 8 minutes. Plunge into cold water and leave until just cool enough to handle.

6 To serve, pour the hot broth into the veggie-filled serving bowls. Peel and halve the eggs, then add two halves to each bowl followed by the crispy tofu. Garnish with the sliced chilli and the coriander leaves.

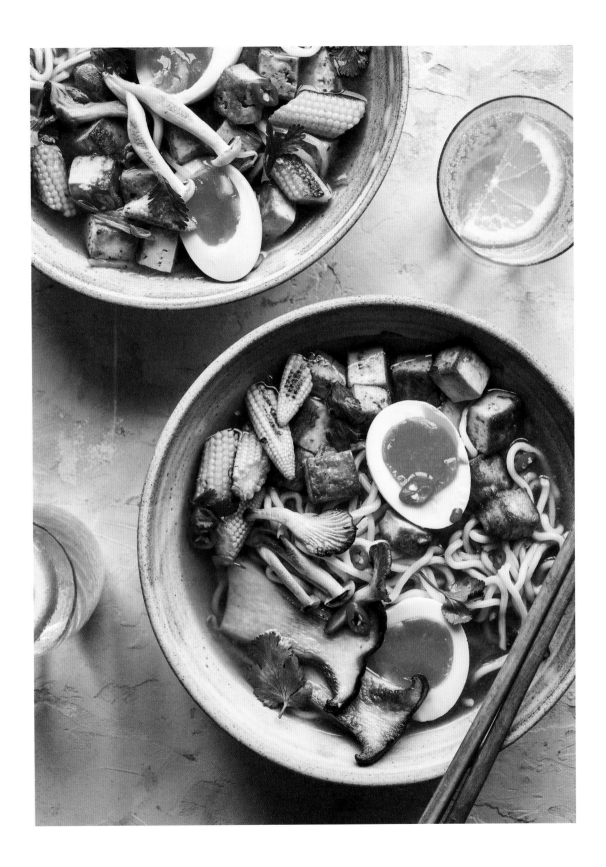

giant couscous, giant flavour salad

Normal couscous is good, but giant couscous is even better! You might see it called pearl or Israeli couscous, but that's the one you want. It cooks more like pasta, but it is such a great carrier of flavour, and this salad is full of that.

2 lemons

2 tsp olive oil

350g cherry tomatoes

1 large courgette, cut into 1cm chunks

A few sprigs of thyme

250g giant couscous

½ red onion, finely sliced

1 red pepper, deseeded and finely diced

100g rocket or baby spinach leaves

A handful of mint leaves, roughly chopped

A small bunch of parsley, roughly chopped

20 pitted black olives, halved

100g feta cheese

2 tbsp extra virgin olive oil

Salt and ground black pepper

1 Preheat the oven to 170°C/150°C fan/Gas Mark 3½. Line a baking tray with greaseproof paper.

2 Take one of the lemons and slice it into rounds, approximately 2-3mm thick. Lay them out on the lined baking tray, drizzle over 1 teaspoon of the olive oil, sprinkle with a pinch of salt and place in the oven.

3 On a separate (unlined) baking tray, add the whole cherry tomatoes and the courgette chunks. Chuck in the thyme sprigs and drizzle with the other teaspoon of olive oil, then give them a pinch of salt and pepper and add to the oven. Let both of these trays roast away for around 20 minutes, until it all starts to colour, then remove and allow to cool, discarding the thyme sprigs.

4 Meanwhile, add the couscous to a pan of lightly salted simmering water and cover. Leave that to cook gently for around 10 minutes, until tender, checking occasionally to ensure there is enough water in the pan. Drain and allow to cool with the veg.

5 To prepare the salad, add the couscous and roasted veg to a large bowl along with any juices from the roasting trays. Add the onion and red pepper along with the rocket or spinach, mint, parsley and olives. Crumble the feta into the bowl.

6 In a separate bowl, whisk together the extra virgin olive oil and the juice of half the remaining lemon (keep the leftover lemon half for another use). Add a pinch or two of salt and pepper and then pour over the salad. Give it all a good mix, then serve.

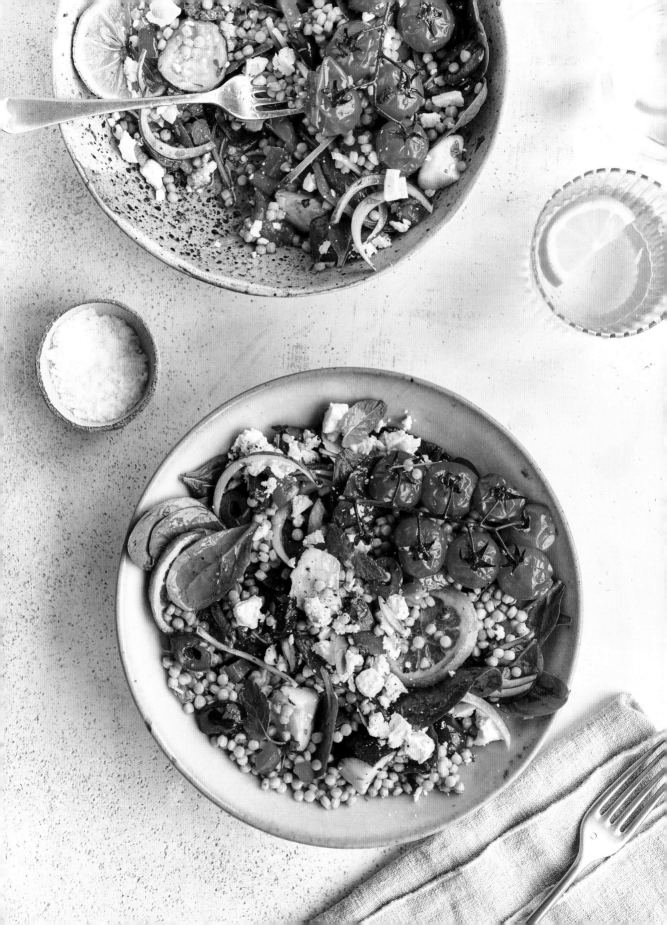

focaccia with pesto and roasted vegetables

serves 8

460kcal per serving

Once you see just how easy this focaccia is, you'll be making it every week! Fresh from the oven and topped with delicious veggies and pesto, you'll wish it was lunchtime all day long.

For the focaccia

2 tsp dried active yeast granules

500ml lukewarm water

2 tsp maple syrup

630g plain flour

1 tbsp salt, plus extra for sprinkling

100ml extra virgin olive oil, plus extra for oiling hands

1 tbsp unsalted butter, softened

For the roasted vegetables

250g cherry tomatoes

4 mixed colour peppers, deseeded and sliced

1½ tbsp olive oil

A sprig of thyme, leaves picked

Salt and ground black pepper

8 tsp green pesto, to serve

1 Prepare the focaccia. Add the yeast to the lukewarm water in a mixing bowl along with the maple syrup and give it a good whisk. Leave to sit for 5-10 minutes, by which time the liquid should look frothy on top. Add the flour and salt to the yeasty liquid, stirring just enough to combine into a dough.

2 Add ½ tablespoon of the extra virgin olive oil into a separate large bowl, then add the dough and turn it in the oil. Cover with clingfilm and leave in the fridge for 24 hours or in a warm place for around 4 hours to allow the dough to more than double in size.

3 When the dough has risen, carefully lift and fold the corners into the middle of the bowl, repeating around each edge of the dough. Do this a few times, to knock the air out and form it into a rough ball.

4 On a large, high-sided rectangular baking tray (approximately 30 x 20cm), add the butter and rub all around the surface, then add 1 tablespoon of the extra virgin olive oil to the tray. Carefully transfer the dough to the tray and turn in the oil, pouring over any oil left in the bowl. Leave the dough to prove, uncovered, in a warm room for around 1½ hours or until it has doubled in size again.

5 Preheat the oven to 220°C/200°C fan/Gas Mark 7.

6 When the dough is ready to bake, if you give it a little press, it should slowly spring back. If it springs back too quickly, leave it for a further 30 minutes. With lightly oiled hands, press your fingers into the dough to create big indentations all over. Drizzle over the remaining extra virgin olive oil and give it a good sprinkle of extra salt. Bake for 20-25 minutes until golden and delicious.

7 While the focaccia bakes, prepare the roasted veg. Add the tomatoes and peppers to a separate baking tray, drizzle with the olive oil and sprinkle with the thyme leaves and some salt and pepper. Add to the oven (on a shelf below the focaccia) and roast for 15–20 minutes (at the same time as the focaccia bakes) or until just starting to caramelise.

8 To serve, cut the hot focaccia into 8 equal-size pieces and split each piece open. Spread 1 teaspoon of pesto over the bottom piece of each pair, top each with some roasted vegetables and then add the focaccia lid.

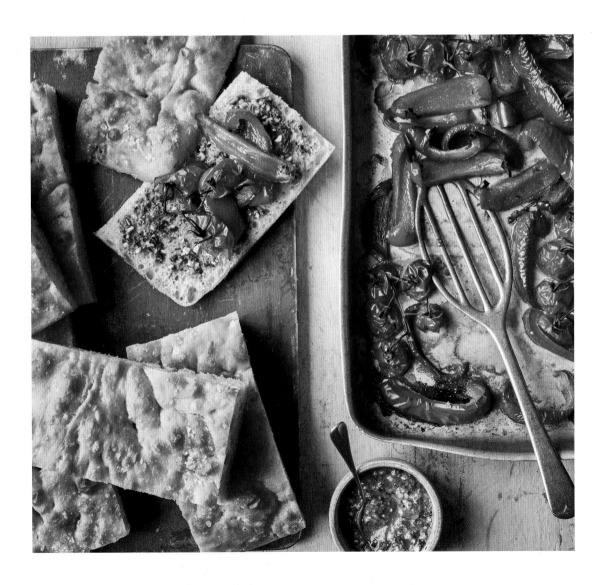

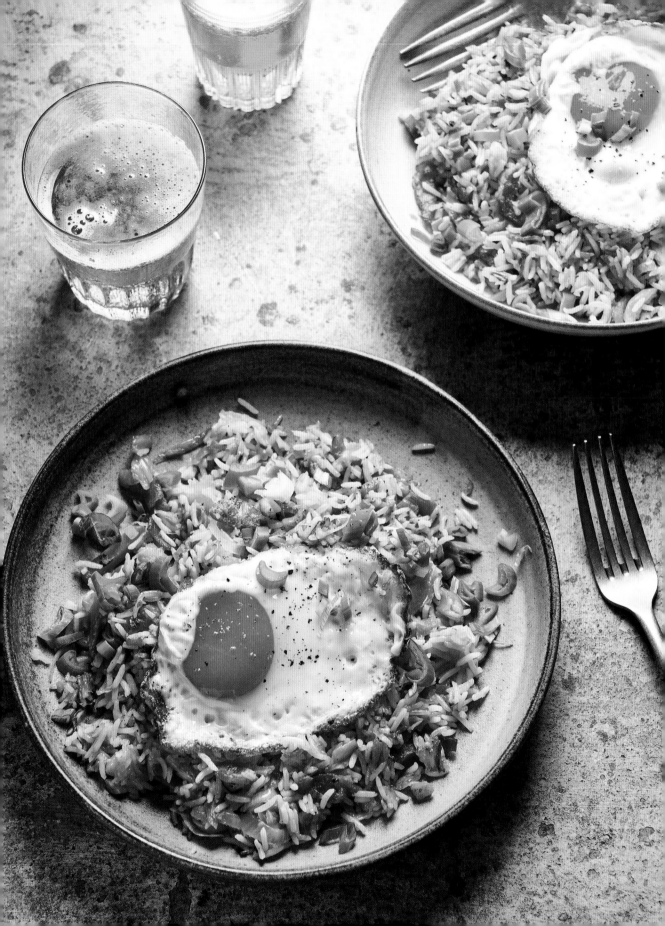

kimchi fried rice

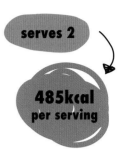

serves 2

485kcal
per serving

In our opinion, this is the best way to use your kimchi! It's one of the most classic of Korean dishes and the perfect brunch. Use pre-cooked rice, either from a packet or use up any leftovers, and you can be eating this in under 10 minutes.

1 tbsp vegetable oil

4 smoked streaky bacon rashers, diced

2 large spring onions, white and green parts separated, thinly sliced

250g cooked basmati rice

240g kimchi (page 229)

2 medium eggs

1 Add half of the oil to a wok or frying pan and place over a medium-high heat. Add in the bacon and fry for a few minutes, so that it just starts to crisp up, then add the white parts of the spring onions. Give it another minute or two and then add in the cooked rice and the kimchi. If you have any juice in the kimchi, add a little of that, too. Stir-fry for a few more minutes so that everything gets nice and hot.

2 While that cooks, add the remaining oil to a separate frying pan and, when hot, crack in the eggs and fry them to your liking.

3 To serve, divide the fried rice between 2 plates, top each portion with a fried egg, then scatter the green parts of the spring onions over the top and serve.

winner's dinners

bacon, pesto mac 'n' three cheese

'I mean, seriously?! You are telling me I can eat this AND still lose weight?!' We hear it all the time, and just remember, #itsfine. That's what we are all about here. Showing you how delicious weight loss can be, and this is just about as delicious as it gets.

250g dried macaroni

30g butter

30g plain flour

350ml semi-skimmed milk

70g mozzarella cheese, grated

70g mature Cheddar cheese, grated

20g green pesto

1 tsp olive oil

100g smoked streaky bacon rashers, diced

25g Parmesan cheese, finely grated

Salt

A few large handfuls of mixed salad leaves, to serve

For smaller appetites, turn this into 5 servings at 460kcal per serving.

1 Preheat the oven to 170°C/150°C fan/Gas Mark 3½.

2 Bring a pan of salted water to the boil, then add the pasta. Give it a good stir and leave it to simmer for 8–9 minutes, until just al dente, then drain.

3 While the pasta cooks, add the butter to a separate saucepan and gently melt, then add the flour and mix well to combine, letting it cook out for a minute or two. Gradually whisk the milk into the pan in batches, starting with small splashes, stirring well to combine each time. It will be a very thick paste at the start and will gradually go lovely and creamy. When all the milk is added, let it simmer gently, stirring regularly, until it has the consistency of double cream.

4 Remove from the heat and add all the mozzarella and all but around 20g of the Cheddar. Add the pesto in as well and give it a good stir so it's well combined, and lovely and stringy and gooey. Stir in the pasta.

5 Pop a small frying pan over a medium heat and add in the oil, then fry the bacon until it gets nice and crisp, around 5 minutes should do it. Add that in to the pasta and sauce, give it one last mix to share that bacon out and then transfer to an ovenproof dish. Top with the remaining Cheddar and all the Parmesan, then bake for 25 minutes until lovely and golden.

6 Serve up with a side salad of mixed leaves and enjoy.

pete's perfect pastitsio

If you like lasagne, then you will love this! We may be biased, but we think this is even better. Not only does this make amazing leftovers for the next couple of days, but if you portion it up and transfer it to the freezer after cooking, you can defrost and reheat it in the oven in 25 minutes and it's an instant 'winner's dinner'!

For the meat sauce

3 tbsp olive oil

2 red onions, finely diced

1 tbsp granulated sugar

A small bunch of thyme, leaves picked

1 large garlic clove, crushed

2 tbsp tomato purée

700g minced beef (5 per cent fat)

75ml red wine

1 x 400g tin chopped tomatoes

1 tsp ground cinnamon

2 beef stock cubes

2 bay leaves

For the pasta

260g dried bucatini pasta

1 tbsp olive oil

2 medium eggs, beaten

180g halloumi cheese, grated

A good handful of parsley, chopped

For the white sauce

80g butter

80g plain flour

700ml semi-skimmed milk

1 Preheat the oven to 170°C/150°C fan/Gas Mark 3½.

2 To make the meat sauce, add the oil to a large frying pan over a medium heat. Add the onions along with the sugar and a tablespoon of the thyme leaves. Fry gently for 5 minutes before stirring in the garlic. Cook for a further 1–2 minutes before adding the tomato purée, then fry for a further couple of minutes.

3 Add the minced beef and do your best to break it up so you don't have any large lumps. Cook until browned all over (about 5–8 minutes), then add the wine and increase the heat. Let that bubble away until the liquid has been absorbed, then add the tomatoes, cinnamon, crumbled stock cubes and bay leaves. Drop the heat down to a simmer and leave the sauce to bubble away, uncovered, for 15 minutes while you prepare the rest.

4 Cook the pasta according to the packet instructions, draining it a couple of minutes before the end of the recommended cooking time. Brush the oil around a large baking dish and add the drained pasta along with the eggs, halloumi and parsley. Give it all a good mix to combine.

5 For the white sauce, place a medium saucepan over a medium heat and add the butter. Allow it to melt without catching, then add the flour and whisk well to combine, cooking it out for a couple of minutes. Add the milk, in small amounts at the start, whisking continuously. As the sauce thickens, add more milk until it is all combined and the sauce is smooth with the consistency of double cream. Remove from the heat, add the nutmeg and all but

½ tsp grated nutmeg

80g Parmesan cheese, finely grated

3 medium egg yolks

Salt and ground black pepper

A few large handfuls of mixed salad leaves, to serve

For smaller appetites, turn this into 10 servings at 500kcal per serving.

1 tablespoon of the Parmesan along with a good pinch of salt and pepper. Finally, whisk in the egg yolks until combined.

6 Remove the bay leaves from the meat sauce, add in one large ladleful of the white sauce and stir well to combine. Pour all the meat sauce over the pasta, evenly distributing it, then cover with the remaining white sauce. Sprinkle over the remaining Parmesan.

7 Bake for 30–40 minutes until golden and bubbling. Remove from the oven and leave to rest for 5 minutes before serving with some salad leaves on the side.

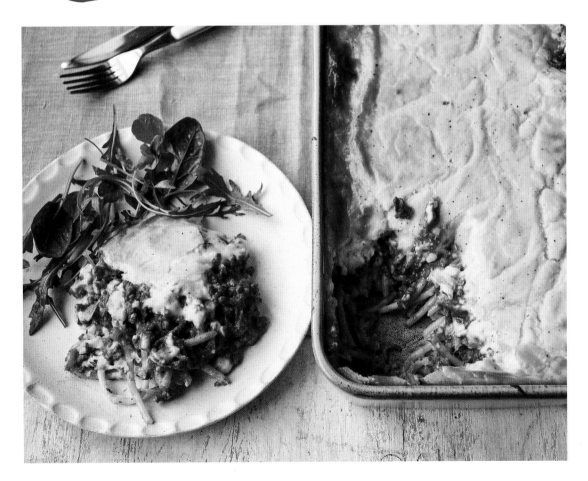

the 'no washing-up' chicken fajita festival

The ultimate weeknight meal here. Not only can it be prepared in around 20 minutes, but it's also all done in the one baking tray. And, if you line that with greaseproof paper, you don't even need to wash that up!

3 mixed colour peppers, deseeded and thinly sliced

2 large red onions, thinly sliced

700g boneless, skinless chicken breasts, thinly sliced

4 tsp olive oil

3 tbsp fajita seasoning

12 small tortillas

A small bunch of coriander

2 limes, cut into quarters

100ml soured cream

60g Cheddar cheese, grated

For smaller appetites, turn this into 6 servings at 435kcal per serving.

1 Preheat the oven to 180°C/160°C fan/Gas Mark 4. Line a large baking tray with greaseproof paper.

2 Add the peppers, red onions and chicken to the lined baking tray, then mix the oil with the fajita seasoning in a small bowl. Pour the oil mix over the chicken and vegetables and then get your hands in there to give it a good mix, so that everything gets coated. Spread it all out in an even layer on the tray. Bake for 15-20 minutes or until the chicken is golden and the vegetables are soft.

3 While that cooks, prepare the extras. Wrap the tortillas in foil and pop those in the oven for the last 5 minutes of the cooking time, so they get lovely and warm.

4 Rip the coriander leaves away from the stalks, discarding the stalks, and have those ready along with the quartered limes, soured cream and Cheddar.

5 When everything is ready, you know what to do! Just pile it all into the tortillas and enjoy.

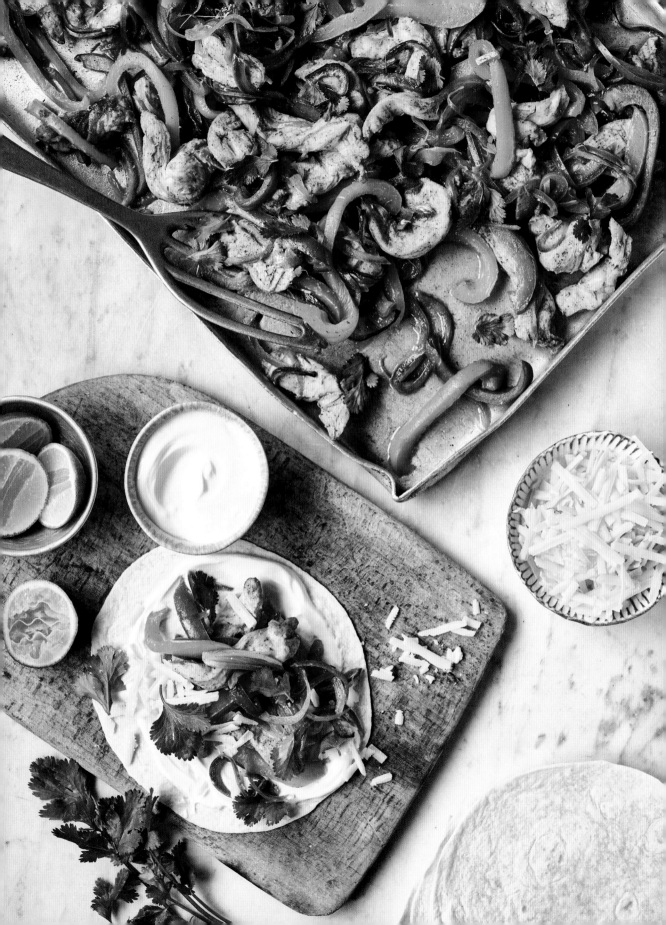

four fish in the dish pie

If you're a fish fan, this one is classic comfort food. And if you aren't, well maybe this is the meal to change that! As a nation, we don't eat enough fish and it has so many amazing health benefits that we really should get it in us a bit more often.

540kcal per serving

750g white potatoes, peeled and roughly chopped

55g unsalted butter

40g plain flour

600ml semi-skimmed milk

180g skinless smoked haddock fillet, cut into bite-sized pieces

180g skinless salmon fillet, cut into bite-sized pieces

125g raw small scallops (shells removed)

200g raw peeled prawns

2 tbsp tartare sauce

100g samphire

Salt and ground black pepper

For smaller appetites, turn this into 5 servings at 435kcal per serving.

1 Preheat the oven to 180°C/160°C fan/Gas Mark 4.

2 Get the mash on the go by adding the potatoes to a pan of salted boiling water. Leave those to bubble away for 20 minutes or until soft enough to mash, then drain and leave to steam-dry.

3 While the spuds cook, add all but 1 tablespoon of the butter to a separate saucepan over a medium heat and leave it to melt. When almost melted, add the flour and start to whisk to combine until you get a thick paste. Add the milk in batches (keeping back 50ml for the mash). Start with a few splashes and work up. After each addition of milk, whisk the mix so that it thickens. At the start it will turn into a big lump straight away, but as you add more milk it will get lovely and thick and creamy. When you have added all the milk and the sauce is lump-free and piping hot, remove from the heat.

4 Now it's just a case of piling all the fish and seafood into the white sauce, then give that all a good stir to combine. Transfer the mix to an ovenproof dish.

5 Give the cooked spuds a good mashing, making sure you get rid of any lumps. Add the remaining milk and butter, the tartare sauce and a good pinch of salt and pepper, then beat the mix to combine. When it's lovely and creamy, spoon lumps of the mash over the fish mix, then smooth them out with a fork to cover the whole dish. Bake for 30–40 minutes until you get that perfect crispy top.

6 For the samphire, add it to a pan of boiling water and cook for 2–3 minutes, then drain. For each portion, serve some samphire alongside a big spoonful of the fish pie.

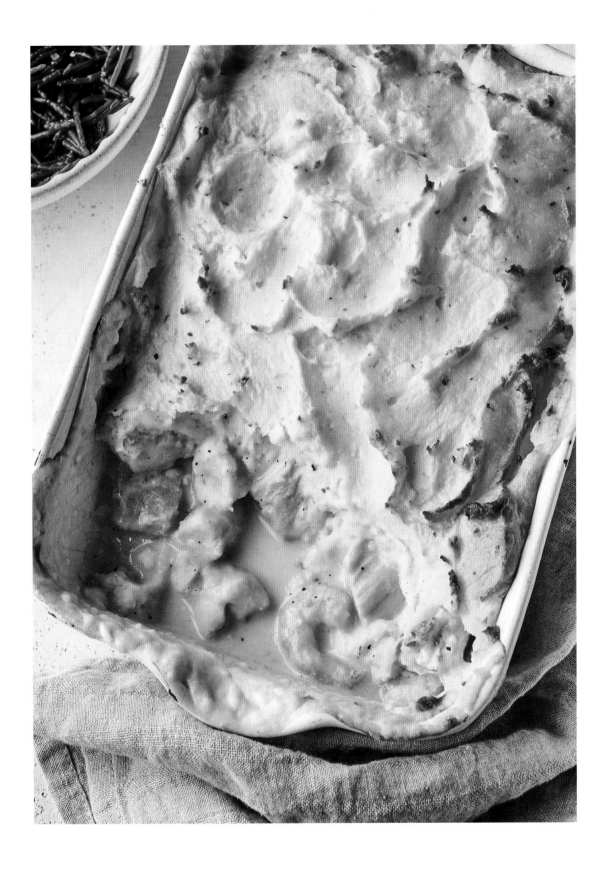

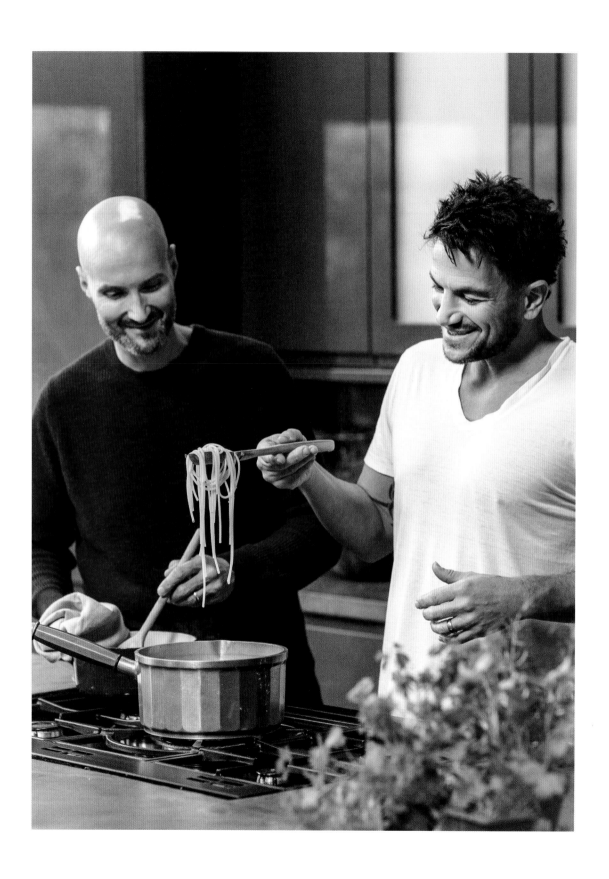

sensational sausage and fennel ragù

This super quick meal is the perfect weeknight feast. Using ready-made sausages means you get a real flavour punch without having to worry about too many spices and herbs, and the sauce couldn't be any easier to knock up.

2 tsp olive oil

2 red onions, finely diced

3 garlic cloves, finely diced

A good pinch of dried chilli flakes (or to taste)

1 tsp fennel seeds

3 tsp dried Italian herb seasoning

6 good-quality pork sausages

3 tsp tomato purée

1 x 400g tin chopped tomatoes

½ chicken stock cube

250g dried spaghetti

4 tsp Parmesan cheese, finely grated

A handful of parsley, roughly chopped (optional)

Salt and ground black pepper

1 Place a large frying pan over a medium heat and add the oil. When hot, add the onions and fry gently for 5 minutes, stirring regularly to ensure they don't colour. Stir in the garlic, chilli flakes, fennel seeds and dried herbs.

2 Remove the skins from the sausages and add the meat into the pan along with the tomato purée. Using a wooden spoon, break up the sausagemeat to make it as chunky or smooth as you like, and let that fry away for another 5 minutes.

3 Now it's just a case of adding in the tomatoes and the crumbled stock cube along with a splash of water and a good pinch of salt and pepper. Stir to combine, then cover with a foil (or pan) lid and leave to simmer gently for 20 minutes.

4 While that bubbles away, cook the pasta according to the packet instructions, then drain. When everything is ready, serve the sausage ragù over the pasta and top with the Parmesan and parsley (if using).

Top Tip: Making it for fewer than 4 (or 5) people? Just cook enough pasta for the number of servings you are making, then pop any excess sausage ragù into a freezerproof container and stash it in the freezer for an even quicker weeknight meal. It will keep in the freezer for up to 6 months. Defrost, then reheat until piping hot to serve.

For smaller appetites, turn this into 5 servings at 480kcal per serving.

say 'aloo' to john's favourite curry

This Indian dish known as Aloo Keema took us by storm and quickly became John's go-to spicy option.

serves 4

660kcal per serving

For smaller appetites, turn this into 6 servings at 440kcal per serving.

For the curry

2 tbsp vegetable oil

2 red onions, diced

4 garlic cloves, finely diced

2.5cm piece of fresh root ginger, peeled and finely diced

1 x 400g tin chopped tomatoes

2 tsp ground coriander

2 tsp ground cumin

1 tsp chilli powder (or to taste)

½ tsp garam masala

1 tsp paprika

400g minced lamb (lean)

2 medium white potatoes, peeled and thinly sliced

A small handful of coriander, chopped

Salt and ground black pepper

For the chapatis

140g plain wholemeal flour

140g plain white flour, plus extra for dusting

1 tsp salt

2 tbsp vegetable oil, plus extra for cooking

About 200ml hot water

1 For the curry, add the oil to an ovenproof casserole and fry the onions, garlic and ginger over a low heat for around 5 minutes. Add the chopped tomatoes and all the spices along with a good couple of pinches of salt and pepper.

2 Leave the sauce to bubble away for 5 minutes, breaking up any big chunks of tomato with a spoon. Stir in the minced lamb and cook for a further 5 minutes before adding 200ml of water. Cover, bring to the boil, then leave to simmer over a medium heat for 30 minutes.

3 When the sauce is lovely and thick, add in the sliced potatoes and drop the heat to low. Cover and leave to cook for a final 10–15 minutes, to allow the spuds to soften. Stir through the chopped coriander to finish.

4 Meanwhile, make the chapatis. Add the flours and salt to a bowl and combine, then add the oil and stir in with just enough hot water to get the dough to combine but not become too sticky.

5 Add a little flour to a board/work surface and knead the dough for around 10 minutes, until smooth and elastic. Divide into 12 pieces and roll each piece into a ball, then leave them to rest for 5 minutes.

6 On the floured board/surface, roll each ball out until nice and thin (approximately 15cm across), aiming to create something similar to a tortilla. Lightly oil a frying pan and heat over a medium-high heat until hot and smoking, then pop a chapati into the pan (cook them one at a time) and cook for around 30 seconds on each side, to get a little colour on it. Keep the cooked chapatis hot in a low oven while you cook the rest in the same way. Serve the curry with the hot chapatis to accompany.

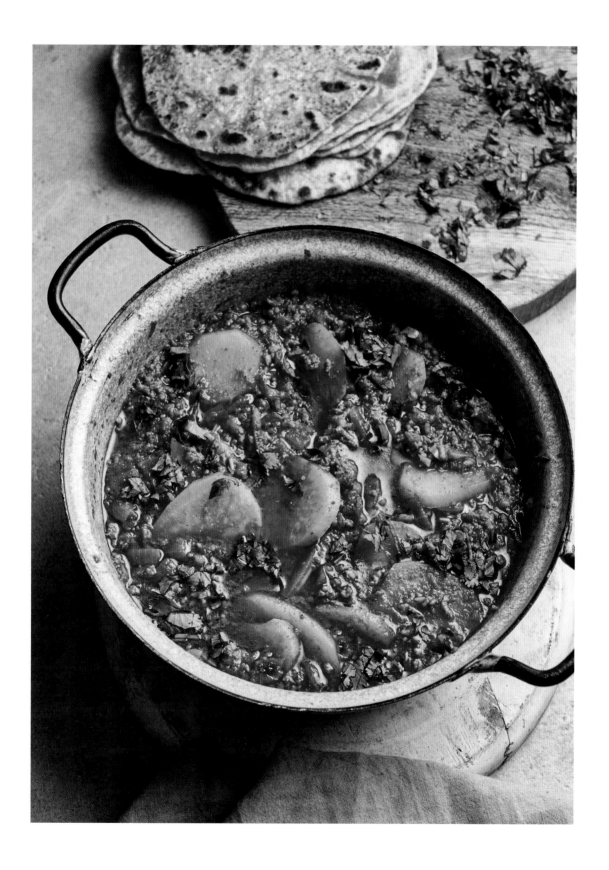

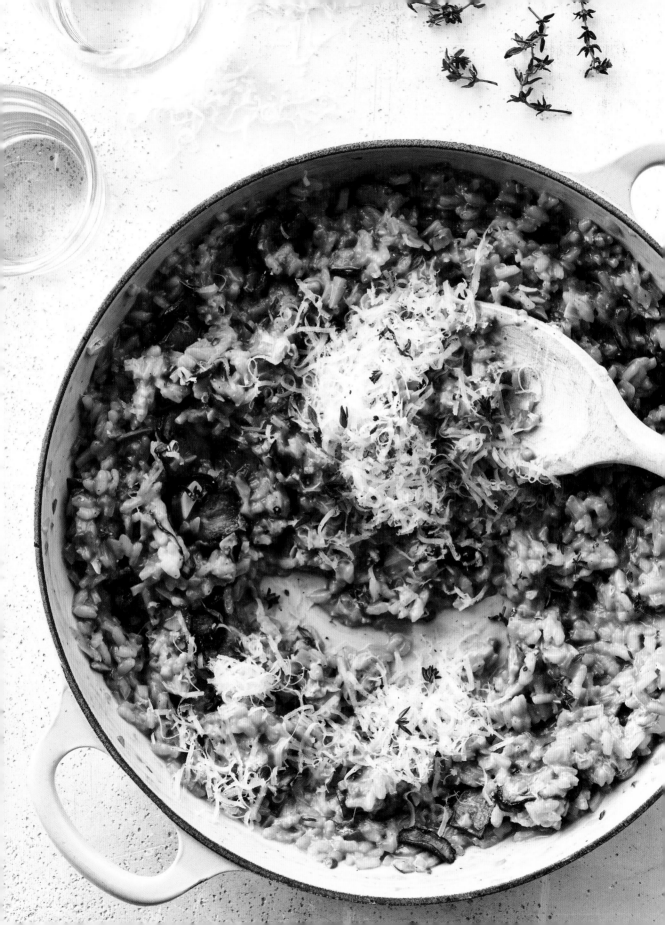

the fun guys risotto

Don't be put off when you see the word risotto. The way some people talk about it, you would think you need a degree to be able to cook it! But it's just a case of taking it one step at a time.

1 litre boiling water

2 vegetable stock cubes

15g dried porcini mushrooms

1 tbsp olive oil

1 large white onion, diced

1 garlic clove, minced

A few sprigs of thyme, leaves picked

200g chestnut mushrooms (150g diced, 50g sliced)

150g risotto rice

70ml white wine

2 tbsp single cream

30g Parmesan cheese, finely grated

10g butter

Salt and ground black pepper

serves 3

350kcal per serving

1 Add the boiling water to a large saucepan, then crumble in the stock cubes and add the porcini mushrooms. Simmer the mushrooms gently until soft, about 5-10 minutes, then remove with a slotted spoon, chop and reserve. Keep the stock simmering over a low heat.

2 Place a large, high-sided frying pan (or sauté pan) over a medium heat. Add the oil and onion and fry gently for around 5 minutes until starting to soften. Add the garlic and most of the thyme leaves along with a good pinch of salt and pepper. Continue to cook for another 2-3 minutes. Next, in go the diced chestnut mushrooms along with the chopped porcini, give it all a good stir and leave to cook for another 2-3 minutes.

3 Add the rice and stir well to get it all coated in the oil and mushroom mix. Fry for 1-2 minutes more, then stir in the wine and let it boil for a few minutes. Drop the heat back down to medium and start to add the hot stock. Do this in batches, 2 large ladlefuls at a time. Let the liquid get completely absorbed by the rice before you add the next load of stock. Take your time, stirring regularly so you get that lovely creamy texture. It should take around 20-25 minutes in total.

4 When the stock is almost all added, taste the rice. There should be no nuttiness left and the rice should be quite soft. Add the cream and half of the Parmesan, stir well, then remove from the heat. Adjust the seasoning to taste.

5 Place a small pan over a medium heat and add the butter. When melted, add the sliced mushrooms along with the remaining thyme leaves and a pinch of salt and pepper. Let them cook for around 5 minutes, tossing every now and then, until golden and tender.

6 Now it's just a case of stirring a last small ladleful of stock through the risotto, before serving it up topped with the fried sliced mushrooms and a sprinkle of the remaining Parmesan.

all-the-larder enchiladas

Enchiladas – Mexican comfort food at its best! But this one is designed to use up all those bits and bobs you have left over in the fridge.

For the enchilada sauce

1 x 400g tin chopped
   tomatoes

2 tbsp olive oil

2 tsp red wine vinegar

1 tsp chilli powder
   (or to taste)

1 tsp garlic granules

1 tsp ground cumin

A pinch of dried
   chipotle chilli flakes

1 tsp dried oregano

A good pinch of salt

For the enchiladas

1 tbsp olive oil, plus
   extra for drizzling

1 white onion, diced

200g sweet potatoes,
   peeled and cut
   into 1cm cubes

1 large courgette, cut
   into 1cm cubes

1 red pepper, deseeded
   and cut into 1cm cubes

3 garlic cloves,
   finely chopped

A pinch of salt

1 tbsp tomato purée

1 tsp ground cumin

1 tsp ground coriander

1 tsp dried oregano

1 x 400g tin black beans,
   drained and rinsed

A small bunch of
   coriander, chopped

8 small tortillas

80g Cheddar
   cheese, grated

1 Preheat the oven to 170°C/150°C fan/Gas Mark 3½.

2 To make the enchilada sauce, add all the ingredients to a food processor or blender along with 3–4 tablespoons of water, then blitz well until lovely and smooth. Leave to one side.

3 For the enchiladas, place a large frying pan over a medium heat and add the oil. When hot, add the onion and fry gently for 5 minutes, then add the sweet potato, courgette, red pepper and garlic and continue to fry for another 4–5 minutes. Add 3–4 tablespoons of water and the salt and let that bubble away for about 10 minutes until the potato starts to soften.

4 Stir in the tomato purée, spices and oregano, then continue to cook for another 2–3 minutes before removing from the heat. Stir in the black beans along with half of the chopped coriander.

5 In a deep baking tray, around 20 x 30cm, drizzle a little oil and grease well. Add 2–3 tablespoons of the enchilada sauce, spreading it out evenly over the tray. Share out the veg filling across the middle of all 8 tortillas, then roll them up and place, side by side, in the tray. Carefully pour over the rest of the sauce to cover, then sprinkle over the cheese.

6 Cover with foil and bake for 20 minutes, then remove the foil and bake for a further 10 minutes, until hot and bubbling. Serve up with the rest of the chopped coriander sprinkled over.

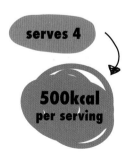

serves 4

500kcal
per serving

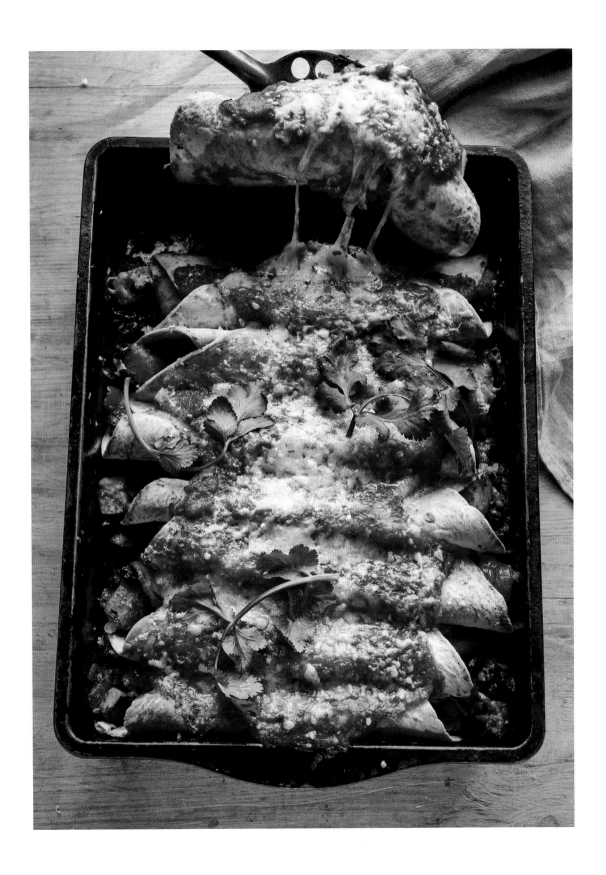

miso-baked asian celeriac

One thing we try to showcase, and particularly to those who steer clear of vegetarian food, is that delicious meals don't have to include meat! And this is the perfect example. In fact, the combination of flavours gives a real sense of meatiness to the celeriac. And it tastes great as well, happy days!

1 tbsp white miso paste

1 tbsp maple syrup

1½ tbsp light soy sauce, plus 2 tsp

1 celeriac

2 tsp vegetable oil

1 pak choi, leaves whole and stalks finely sliced

1 large carrot, cut into thin strips

300g straight-to-wok medium noodles

1 Preheat the oven to 180°C/160°C fan/Gas Mark 4. Line a baking tray with greaseproof paper.

2 Add the miso, maple syrup and the 1½ tablespoons of soy sauce to a bowl. Give it a good mix to break down the miso and make sure everything is well combined.

3 Take the celeriac and cut it into 2 steaks, each around 2–3cm thick. Using a peeler, carefully trim around the edges to get rid of the peel and any lumpy bits. Next, take a sharp knife and carefully cut a criss-cross pattern over one side of each celeriac steak, going approximately halfway through.

4 Place the celeriac slices on to the lined baking tray, criss-cross side up, then add 2 teaspoons of the miso mix to the top of each one. Spread that out over the surface so that it gets an even coating, then pop in the oven. After 10 minutes, remove and add another 2 teaspoons of the miso mix on top of each slice, again spreading it out across the whole surface, then it's back into the oven for another 10 minutes.

5 Finally, switch the oven over to a medium heat grill (or preheat a separate grill to medium) and top the celeriac slices with the remaining miso mix, spreading it out as before. Pop them under the grill for 3–4 minutes, until the sauce is just starting to caramelise.

6 While that all goes on, place a wok over a high heat and add in the veg oil. Pop the sliced pak choi stalks in and stir-fry for a minute or two, then add the leaves, the carrot strips, the noodles and the remaining 2 teaspoons of soy sauce. Continue to stir-fry for another 2–3 minutes to heat everything through, then serve up with the celeriac steaks.

Top Tip: If you have leftover celeriac, don't throw it away! You can blitz it with chicken stock to make a soup; or finely chop it into matchsticks and mix with a little mayonnaise and mustard for a remoulade to serve with fish, or on its own with a little salad.

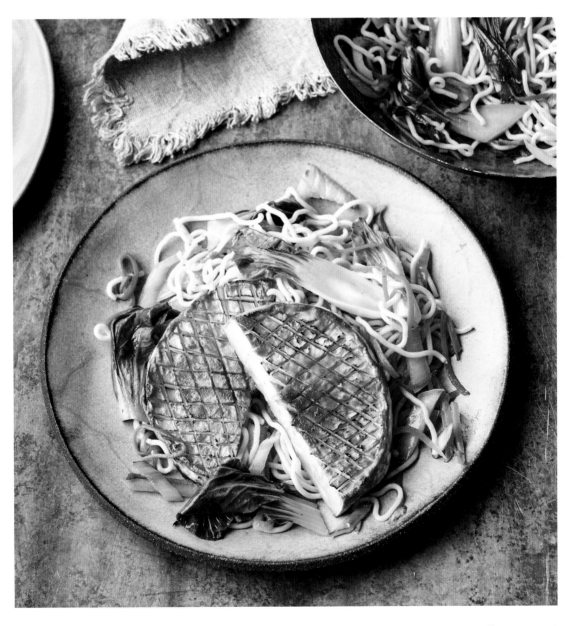

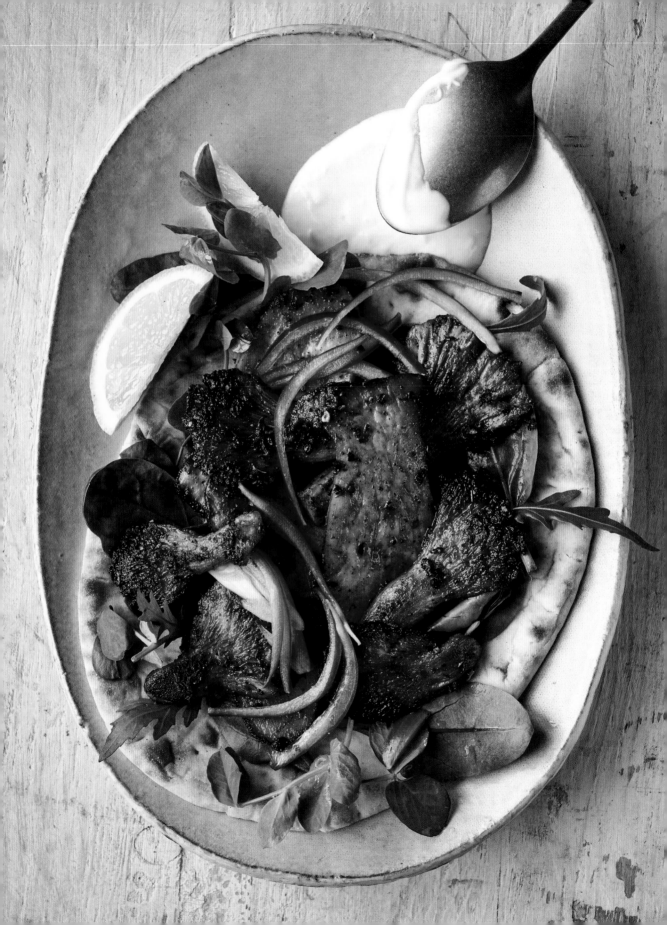

i can't believe it's not chicken kebabs

Every now and then you come across a veggie meal that makes you forget about meat for a moment. This one made us forget about meat for ages, and instead crave these delicious, packed-full-of-flavour mushrooms. And when you combine them with all the other goodies here, well, we could almost go veggie full-time!

½ red onion, thinly sliced
50ml red wine vinegar
1 tsp ground cumin
3 tsp fajita seasoning
2 tsp dried oregano
1 tsp onion granules
½ tsp salt
200g mixed mushrooms
2 tbsp vegetable oil
60g natural yogurt
1 garlic clove, grated
Juice of ½ lemon
2 flatbreads
A large handful of
  salad leaves

1 Start off by making the pickled onions around 2 hours in advance. Place the red onion into a jar, pour in the vinegar and 25ml of water and give them a good press down so all the slices get covered. Seal the lid and leave to one side.

2 Combine the spices, oregano, onion granules and salt in a small bowl. In a large bowl, add the mushrooms, tearing up any really big ones but don't tear them up too much. Add 1 tablespoon of the oil and all the seasoning mix and give the mushrooms a good mix around so they get a coating of everything.

3 Place a large frying pan over a medium heat and add the remaining oil. When hot, add the mushrooms, give them a quick toss around and then place something heavy over them, like a plate, to press them down. Leave to cook for a few minutes, then give them a good stir before covering with the plate again and leaving for another 3-4 minutes. Remove from the pan and roughly slice.

4 For the sauce, just add the yogurt to a bowl, then the garlic and a little squeeze of lemon juice. Give that a good stir.

5 To serve, warm the flatbreads in the oven or as per the packet instructions. Top with the salad leaves and then the mushrooms, before scattering some (drained) pickled onion on top and drizzling over the garlic yogurt.

6 If you weren't already, you are now converted to vegetarian food!

super easy butternut, sage and feta slice

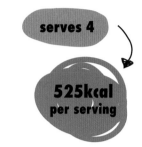

serves 4

525kcal per serving

No stress, no faff, no problem.
The perfect weeknight dinner does exist.

1 small butternut squash, deseeded and cut into rough chunks

1 tsp olive oil

50g feta cheese, crumbled

A few sage leaves, finely chopped

1 red chilli, finely chopped (and deseeded if preferred)

1 x 320g packet chilled fresh ready-rolled puff pastry sheet

2 tsp butter

200g broccoli, broken into florets

Salt and ground black pepper

1 Preheat the oven to 180°C/160°C fan/Gas Mark 4.

2 Toss the butternut chunks in the oil on a baking tray and season with salt and pepper, then spread out in a single layer. Roast for 25 minutes, turning occasionally, until soft and ready to mash.

3 When cooked, pop the squash into a bowl with the feta, sage and chilli. Season with a little more pepper, then mash the lot up until well combined. Leave to cool for 10 minutes.

4 Unroll the sheet of pastry on to a separate baking tray (leave the pastry on the greaseproof paper it comes wrapped in), then spoon the squash mix over one half of the sheet (down the length), leaving a border of around 1cm clear all around the edge. Fold the empty half over the top and then seal the edges with a fork. Melt the butter in a small pan (or in the microwave), then brush it over the slice.

5 Add a few slashes to the top to let the steam escape, then bake for 20–25 minutes until golden brown and crispy.

6 While the slice bakes, cook the broccoli in a pan of lightly salted boiling water for 5 minutes, then drain, and it's all ready to serve.

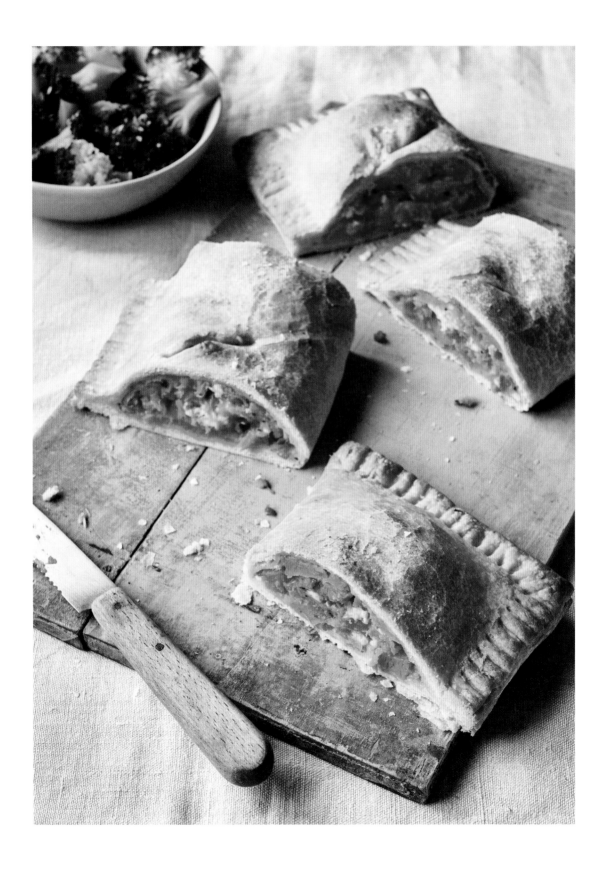

griddled chicken with panzanella

Panzanella might not be something you have heard of before, but it's a classic Italian dish made with slightly stale bread and really ripe tomatoes. It is great on its own, but pairing it up with some griddled chicken breast turns it into a superb main meal that takes very little time to prepare.

For the salad/panzanella

1 tbsp olive oil

150g good-quality, slightly stale bread, cut into 2cm chunks

1 red pepper, deseeded and cut into bite-sized pieces

2 ripe tomatoes, cut into bite-sized pieces

½ red onion, thinly sliced

A few basil leaves, thinly sliced

½ tsp capers, drained and roughly chopped

Salt and ground black pepper

For the dressing

1 small garlic clove, grated

¼ tsp Dijon mustard

2 tsp white wine vinegar

2 tbsp extra virgin olive oil

For the chicken

500g boneless, skinless chicken breasts

½ tbsp dried mixed herbs

1 tbsp olive oil

1 For the salad/panzanella, place a frying pan over a medium heat and add the olive oil. When hot, add the bread chunks with a pinch of salt. Let those crisp up – cook for around 10 minutes, tossing every now and then, until lovely and golden.

2 When they're ready, add the toasted bread cubes to a large bowl along with the red pepper, tomatoes, onion, basil and capers. Season with a pinch of salt and pepper.

3 Add the dressing ingredients into a small bowl along with a further pinch of salt and pepper and give them a really good whisk, until you get a lovely smooth texture. Pour over the salad and gently mix to ensure everything gets coated. Leave to one side.

4 For the chicken, lay the breast pieces in between some clingfilm and give them a bash to make the pieces all the same thickness. Sprinkle over the mixed herbs, a little salt and pepper and the olive oil, then toss to make sure they get a good coating all over. If you have a griddle pan, get that nice and hot over a medium-high heat. If not, a normal frying pan is just as good.

5 Pop the chicken into the hot pan and cook for 4–5 minutes on each side, depending on how thick the pieces are. Make sure they are cooked all the way through with no pink bits, then serve up on top of the delicious salad/panzanella.

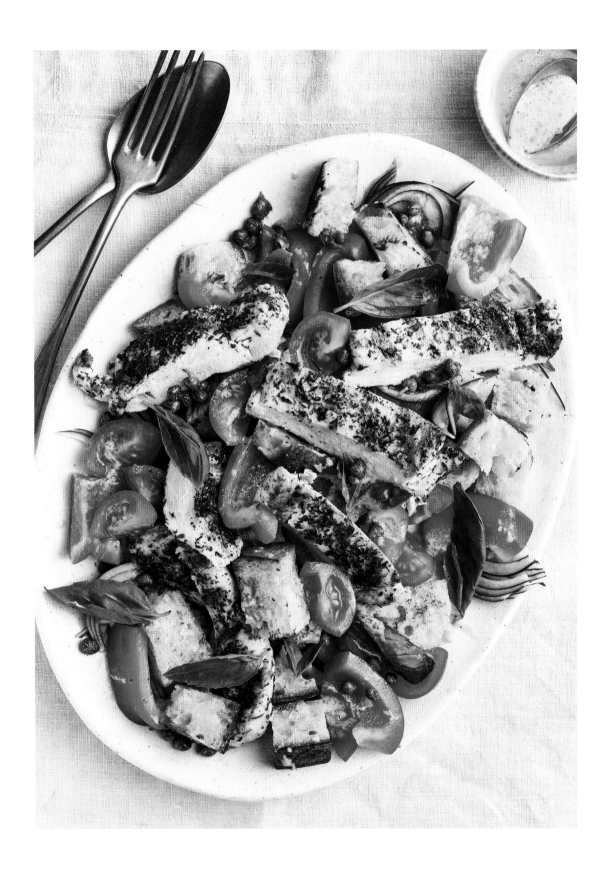

not so guilty pleasures

rocky rice

serves 12

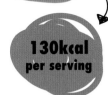

130kcal
per serving

Everyone knows rocky road, right? And those who do also know it can be a bit heavy on the calories. So we wanted to make it a little less so! And we're pretty happy with the result, so hopefully you will be, too.

15g unsalted butter

120g marshmallows (mini marshmallows or larger ones cut into chunks)

100g toasted rice cereal

70g dried cranberries

40g shortbread biscuits, roughly chopped into small chunks

40g dark chocolate, broken into pieces

For smaller appetites, turn this into 16 servings at 100kcal per serving.

1 Line a (roughly) 20cm square cake tin with greaseproof paper.

2 Add the butter to a large saucepan and melt slowly over a medium-low heat. When melted, add the marshmallows and, stirring continuously, allow them to melt until lovely, smooth and gooey.

3 Remove from the heat and add in the rice cereal, cranberries and shortbread pieces. Be quick, as it will start to set as it cools. Pour the rice mix into the lined tin and, using a plastic spatula, press it down so you get a nice even layer. It will get easier to mould and press down as it cools. Leave to one side.

4 To melt the chocolate, pop a small saucepan containing around 5cm of water over a medium heat. Place a heatproof bowl over the pan, making sure it doesn't touch the water below, and add the chocolate to the bowl. Keep an eye on the chocolate as it melts, stirring regularly, and when it's smooth, remove from the heat. Using a spoon, drizzle the chocolate over the top of the rocky rice, making sure you get a good spread.

5 Place in the fridge for about an hour to set and chill. Using a sharp knife, carefully portion up and then tuck in. These will keep in an airtight container in the fridge for up to 3-4 days.

ice cream, three ways

serves 4

Ice cream tastes good, yeah? But that means ice cream is probably bad for you, too, yeah? Well, not when you say #itsfine. And even more so when #itsfine have come up with the recipe!

bananaberry ice cream

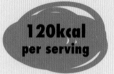
120kcal per serving

180g frozen mixed berries (or use fresh – see step 1)

240g frozen banana chunks (or use fresh – see step 1)

20g maple syrup

80g natural yogurt

1 First thing you need to do with this one is a bit of prep work, if using fresh fruit. Get the fresh berries and peeled banana (cut into chunks) into the freezer at least a couple of hours before you want to make the ice cream (or you can just use ready-frozen berries and banana chunks, if you prefer!).

2 When you are ready to go, pop all the ingredients into a blender and set it off. You want to let this whizz away for a good couple of minutes, to get that lovely creamy texture. It might require a bit of stopping and starting at the beginning, as you push the ingredients around.

3 As with the others here, it's best served straight out of the blender. But if you do freeze it, give it time to start to defrost and then give it a little stir to get the texture back.

mango ice cream

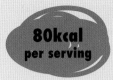

80kcal per serving

300g frozen mango chunks
15g honey
80g natural yogurt

1 It really is this simple. Just pile all the ingredients into a blender and set it off. You want to leave it to really whizz away for a couple of minutes to get that lovely creamy texture. You may also need to scrape down the sides a couple of times to make sure everything gets a good blitz.

2 When smooth and creamy, spoon into serving bowls and tuck in straight away. Or pop it in a suitable container and freeze. Make sure you let it sit out of the freezer for at least 15 minutes before eating.

mint choc chip ice cream

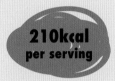

210kcal per serving

25g mint leaves
350g frozen
 banana chunks
200ml light coconut milk
60g dark chocolate chips

1 Pop the mint leaves into a pestle and mortar and give them a really good bash around. You want to turn them into a rough paste, to get all that lovely flavour out.

2 Scrape the mint out into a blender along with the banana and coconut milk and start it up. Let that whizz away until you get that lovely creamy texture, stopping the blender and scraping down the sides as required. When just about combined, add the chocolate chips as well and whizz them through for another few seconds.

3 This is best served straight away when lovely and creamy, but if you do pop it in the freezer, get it out 15 minutes before you want to eat it and give it a good churn with the spoon to get that creaminess back.

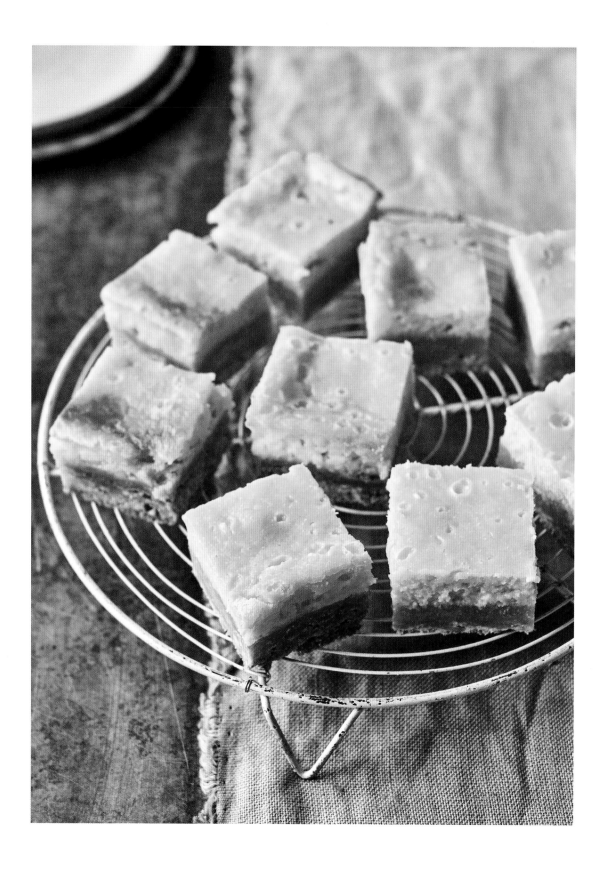

lip-smacking lemon shortcake bites

OK, we know this has a fair bit of refined sugar in it, which isn't ideal all the time. But #itsfine every now and then! So, if you're going to use it, then use it for something really special. And these bars of deliciousness are just that.

For the shortcake base

120g plain flour

50g granulated sugar

110g unsalted butter, cubed

For the cheesecake topping

110g cream cheese (full-fat)

150g granulated sugar

1 tbsp plain flour

90ml freshly squeezed lemon juice

3 large eggs, beaten

½ tsp vanilla extract

For smaller appetites, turn this into 12 servings at 220kcal per serving.

1 Preheat the oven to 170°C/150°C fan/Gas Mark 3½. Line a small square baking tin (approximately 20 x 20cm) with greaseproof paper, making sure the paper goes over the sides to help get the bars out of the tin after baking.

2 To make the base, add the flour, sugar and butter to a bowl and, using your fingertips, work them all together until you get to the texture of fine breadcrumbs. Transfer to the lined baking tin, then press the crumb mixture down so you get an even layer across the bottom and about 2.5cm up the sides of the tin. Pop that in the oven and bake for 10 minutes.

3 While that cooks, make the topping. Add the cream cheese and sugar to a bowl and beat together until smooth and creamy. Mix in the flour, lemon juice, eggs and vanilla, making sure you combine it all well.

4 When the crumb base comes out of the oven, pour over the cheesecake mix, then pop it back in the oven for another 20–25 minutes. You want the topping to be just set and to see some dark patches appear on the top.

5 Remove from the oven and leave to cool in the tin for an hour outside the fridge and then for another hour in the fridge. It should now be set and easy to remove from the tin and portion up. Enjoy!

delicious doughnuts

makes 12 small ring doughnuts

85kcal per serving

Who doesn't love a good doughnut? And we know by now that there's no reason to feel any guilt after eating one. But in case you aren't sure yet, we wanted to help by making these delicious baked doughnuts. You just need to invest in a small doughnut tray and then choose which of the amazing toppings you prefer!

120g plain flour
70g granulated sugar
1 tsp baking powder
A pinch of salt
30g unsalted butter, melted
1 large egg
80ml semi-skimmed milk
1 tsp vanilla extract
Vegetable oil, for greasing

1 Preheat the oven to 170°C/150°C fan/Gas Mark 3½.

2 Add the flour, sugar, baking powder and salt to a bowl and mix to combine. In a separate bowl, whisk together the melted butter, the egg, milk and vanilla extract. Next, simply pour the wet ingredients into the dry and stir just enough to combine and remove any floury lumps.

3 Wet your finger with a little vegetable oil and give each mould in a 12-cup doughnut tray a light greasing. Half-fill the moulds with the doughnut batter to allow room for the doughnuts to rise while cooking.

4 Bake for 10 minutes, until lovely and golden. Let them cool in the tray for a few minutes before carefully removing and leaving them on a wire rack to cool completely. Serve with the topping of your choice (see below).

cinnamon sugar

tops 12 small doughnuts

95kcal per serving

1 tbsp granulated sugar
½ tsp ground cinnamon

1 Mix the sugar and cinnamon together in a small bowl. As soon as you can handle the warm doughnuts, give them a dip and a press into the cinnamon sugar. Once you have dipped and covered them all, any excess sugar you have left can just be sprinkled over the top.

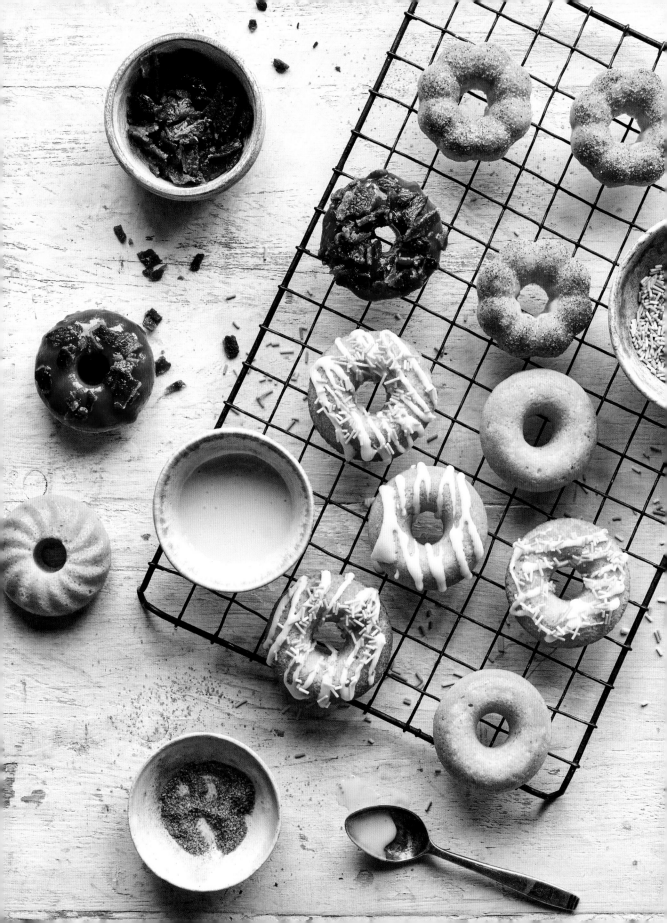

vanilla frosted with sprinkles

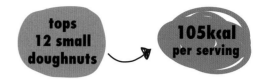

40g icing sugar
¼ tsp vanilla extract
½ tbsp semi-
  skimmed milk
10g sprinkles

1 Add the icing sugar, vanilla and milk to a small bowl and give it a really good mix, so all the sugar is combined. Carefully dip the tops of each cooled doughnut into the frosting or alternatively drizzle it over, then scatter them with the sprinkles.

salted caramel and candied bacon

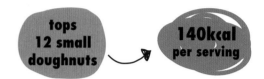

½ tbsp light soft
  brown sugar
½ tsp white wine vinegar
1 tsp maple syrup
75g smoked streaky
  bacon rashers
50g granulated sugar
25g unsalted butter,
  cut into small cubes
30ml single cream
¼ tsp salt

1 Preheat the oven to 170°C/150°C fan/Gas Mark 3½.

2 Add the brown sugar, vinegar and maple syrup to a small bowl and mix well to combine. Set aside.

3 Place the bacon rashers on a wire rack set over a baking tray and pop in the oven for 10 minutes. Remove and baste with the maple syrup mix on both sides and then put back in the oven for 5 minutes. Repeat this twice, making sure you have used up all the maple syrup mix, giving it one last 5-minute blast in the oven (30 minutes cooking time in total). The bacon should be dark and sticky, but it will be hot, so leave it for a few minutes to cool down.

4 Now make the caramel. This really does get hot, so be careful. Place a heavy-based saucepan over a medium heat and add the granulated sugar. When that starts to melt, make sure you are continuously stirring with a wooden spoon as it will burn easily. When completely melted and light brown, add the butter. It will foam away, but keep carefully stirring. When the butter has been incorporated, slowly and carefully add the cream while stirring. When all the cream is in, let it bubble away for another minute or two, then remove from the heat and stir through the salt.

5 Let the caramel cool down – it will get a little thicker as it does. You can then drizzle it over the warm or cold doughnuts before breaking the candied bacon into pieces and scattering across the top.

oatmeal raisin cookie cakes

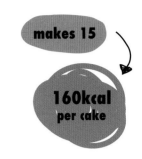

Are they a cookie? Are they a cake? (Are they even a biscuit?!) We aren't sure what you classify them as, but we do know they taste amazing. And with zero refined sugar in there, they are pretty special, too!

100g plain flour
200g porridge oats
1 tsp bicarbonate of soda
1 tsp ground mixed spice
A pinch of salt
100g butter, melted
100g maple syrup
1 large egg
1 tsp vanilla extract
50g raisins

1 Preheat the oven to 170°C/150°C fan/Gas Mark 3½. Line 1 large or 2 smaller baking trays with greaseproof paper.

2 In a large bowl, add the flour, oats, bicarbonate of soda, mixed spice and salt. Give that a good whisk together.

3 In a separate bowl, add the melted butter, the maple syrup, egg and vanilla and give that a good whisk as well.

4 Now it's just a case of adding the wet ingredients to the dry, then mixing until there aren't any floury bits left. Finally, chuck in the raisins and fold them through.

5 Dollop golf ball-sized lumps on to the lined baking tray(s), pressing them down a little to flatten them out, leaving about a 2cm gap in between each ball (you'll make about 15 in total).

6 Pop them in the oven for 8-10 minutes, until lovely and golden. Transfer to a wire rack and leave to cool, then serve or store in an airtight container for up to 3-4 days.

four-ingredient fudgy brownies

serves 8

105kcal per serving

Who knew something this delicious could come from just four ingredients! Egg-free, gluten-free and with no butter, they work for just about any allergy or dietary preference you could have.

200g bananas (peeled)
65g tahini
4 tsp unsweetened cocoa powder
20g milk chocolate chips

1 Preheat the oven to 190°C/170°C fan/Gas Mark 5. Grab yourself a baking tin (about 20 x 15cm) and line it with greaseproof paper.

2 In a large bowl, give the bananas a really good mashing with a fork, until you get a reasonably smooth paste. Add all the other ingredients and stir well to combine.

3 Pour the mixture into the lined tin and smooth over to get a nice even layer, then bake for 15-20 minutes, depending on the thickness of the layer. You want the brownie to feel a little soft when it comes out of the oven.

4 Leave it to cool slightly in the tin and then portion up and remove. Either serve warm, or cool and then chill in the fridge before serving. We think they taste better out of the fridge, but they are also very tasty fresh from the oven! These will keep in an airtight container in the fridge for up to 3-4 days.

Top Tip: If you're allergic to sesame seeds, you can replace the tahini with the same amount of smooth peanut butter, dropping the calories to 100kcal per serving.

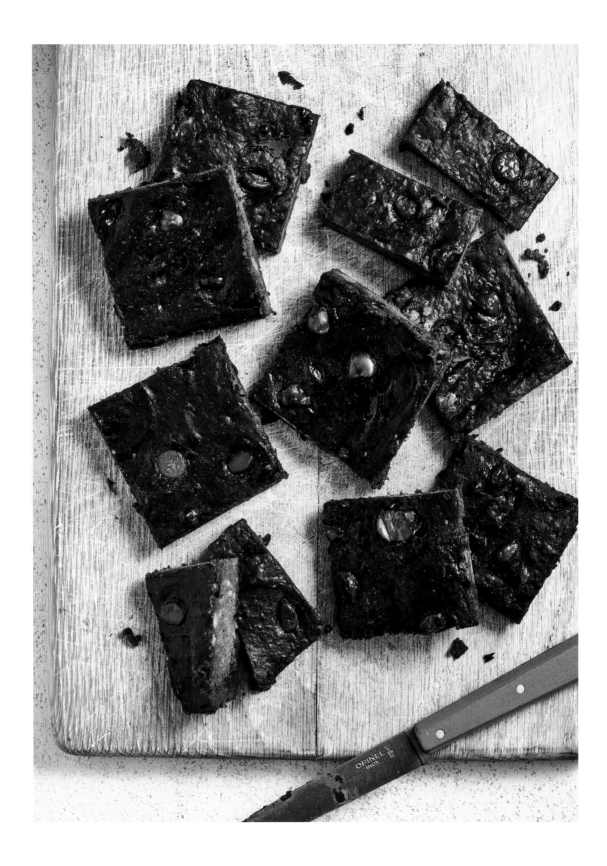

protein bites, three ways

Getting a hit of protein into your day doesn't have to be from a boring shake. These three options are not only super quick to knock up but far tastier, and will last in an airtight container in the fridge for 3–4 days.

carrot cake bites

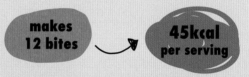

makes 12 bites → 45kcal per serving

50g pitted dates, roughly torn
25g raisins
Boiling water, to cover
50g carrot, grated
40g porridge oats
30g protein powder
½ tsp ground mixed spice

1 Place the dates and raisins into a bowl and just cover with the boiling water. Leave them to soak for 5 minutes.

2 Remove the fruit from the bowl, reserving the liquid, and add the fruit to a food processor along with all the other ingredients. Set it off and let it whizz away, stopping the machine every now and then to scrape down the sides. Add a little of the reserved soaking water to help the mix come together but do this very gradually, you don't want to make it too wet.

3 When you can roll the mix up into balls that hold, but aren't really sticky, that's the perfect texture. Divide and roll the mix into 12 equal-size balls. Serve or store in an airtight container in the fridge for up to 3-4 days.

Top Tip: Don't fancy using the protein powder? Just leave it out and add a little less liquid to the mix, taking the calories down to 35kcal per bite.

cookie dough bites

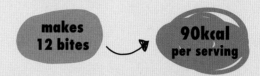

makes 12 bites → 90kcal per serving

100g tahini
50g protein powder
1 tbsp natural yogurt
1 tsp maple syrup
½ tsp vanilla extract
30g dark chocolate chips

1 Add the tahini, protein powder, yogurt, maple syrup and vanilla to a bowl and give it a really good beating. You want to get that lovely texture of cookie dough, kind of crumbly and kind of sticky. When you get to that, add the chocolate chips in and just stir again enough to combine them.

2 Using slightly wet hands, roll up small balls of the mix, aiming to get 12 equal-size bites. Serve or store in an airtight container in the fridge for up to 3-4 days.

Top Tip: Don't fancy using the protein powder? Just swap for the same amount of ground flaxseeds and use 1 teaspoon of vanilla extract instead, taking the calories to 95kcal per bite.

white chocolate and raspberry bites

makes 14 bites → 90kcal per serving

70g tahini
30g protein powder
30g ground almonds
60g porridge oats
20g honey
2 tbsp natural yogurt
2 tbsp freeze-dried raspberries
30g white chocolate chips

1 Line a small baking tray with greaseproof paper.

2 Get the tahini, protein powder, ground almonds, oats, honey and yogurt into a food processor and set that off. Let it whizz away until you get a mixture that you can form into a ball, then add the freeze-dried raspberry pieces and fold them through the mix. Roll into balls, aiming for around 14, then place to one side.

3 Pop a small saucepan over a low-medium heat and add around 2-3cm of boiling water. Place a heatproof bowl over the top, making sure that it doesn't touch the water below, then add the chocolate chips to the bowl. Let them melt, stirring occasionally, until lovely and glossy, then remove from the heat.

4 Carefully dip one side of each ball into the chocolate, then place on to the lined baking tray. When all the bites have been dipped, pop them in the fridge to let the chocolate set. Serve or store in an airtight container in the fridge for up to 3-4 days.

Top Tip: Don't fancy using the protein powder? Just add 30g of ground flaxseeds in its place, taking the calories to 95kcal per bite.

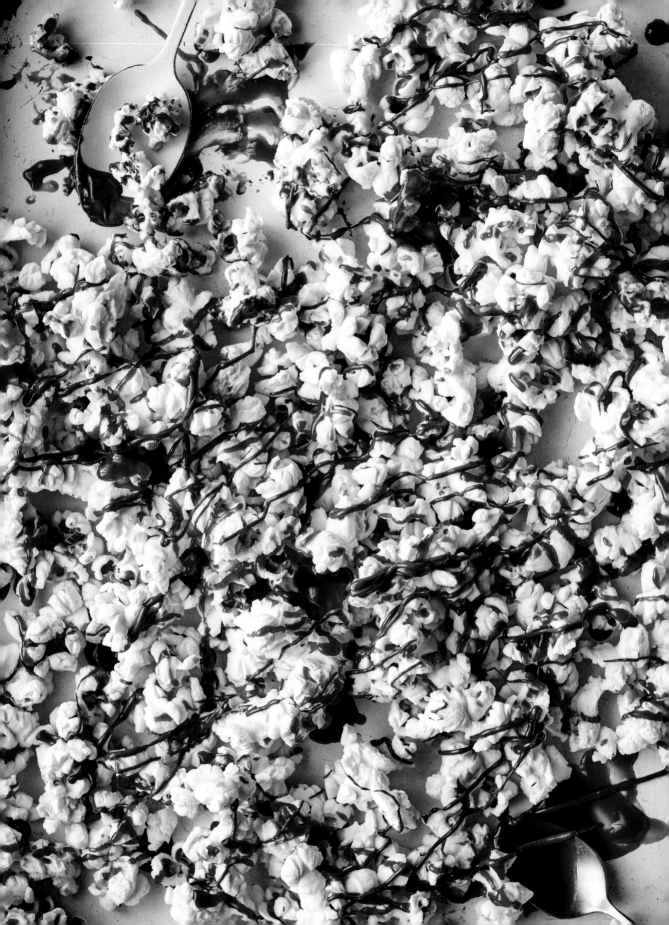

you will roll-o over for this popcorn

This recipe was one of those moments where you really hit the jackpot. We had leftover ingredients that were perfect for making the caramel and a few chocolate chips in the cupboard and this is the result!

For the caramel (makes 12 servings)

60g light soft brown sugar

2 tbsp unsalted butter

40ml single or double cream

For the popcorn

30g milk chocolate chips

50g popcorn kernels

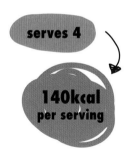

serves 4

140kcal per serving

1 This recipe provides enough for 12 servings of caramel, but you will only need a third of what you make for the 4 servings of popcorn in this recipe. The rest can be stored in an airtight container in the fridge for up to a few days, or in the freezer for a few months. Once defrosted (or chilled), reheat in the microwave on High for around 40–60 seconds.

2 To make the caramel, place a heavy-based saucepan over a medium heat and add the sugar. As it melts, make sure you are continuously stirring with a wooden spoon, as it will burn easily. When completely melted, add the butter. It will foam away, but keep carefully stirring. When the butter has been incorporated, slowly and carefully add the cream while stirring. When all the cream is in, let it bubble away for another minute, then remove from the heat and place to one side.

3 For the popcorn, place a small saucepan over a low-medium heat and add around 2.5cm of boiling water. Place a heatproof bowl over the top, making sure that it doesn't touch the water below, then add the chocolate chips to the bowl. Let them melt, stirring occasionally, until lovely and glossy, then remove from the heat.

4 Finally, add the popcorn kernels to a microwaveable bowl and cover with a suitable plate (or lid). Place in the microwave and heat on High for 4–5 minutes, until you stop hearing popping. Empty the popcorn into a bowl, removing any unpopped kernels.

5 Take the melted chocolate and the caramel and start drizzling. Make it as neat or as messy as you like, it will taste as good either way! This is best enjoyed freshly made.

eating out, but eating in

kentucky fine chicken

serves 2

570kcal
per serving

We're all for a trip to see the Colonel every now and then, but you don't have to rely on him for your chicken burger cravings! Our version is so simple to prepare, but is as good as the real thing, and a lot cheaper as well.

For the chicken

300g boneless, skinless chicken breasts (try and get 2 breast portions roughly the same size)

½ tbsp plain flour

2 tsp Cajun seasoning

1 medium egg

45g panko breadcrumbs

1 tsp olive oil

For the coleslaw

1 small carrot, peeled and grated

40g red cabbage, grated

½ red onion, thinly sliced

2 tbsp natural yogurt

2 tsp mayonnaise (page 231)

½ tsp American mustard

Salt and ground black pepper

To serve

2 brioche burger buns, split in half

2 pickled gherkins, drained and sliced

1 Preheat the oven to 170°C/150°C fan/Gas Mark 3½. Line a baking tray with greaseproof paper.

2 Place the chicken breasts between 2 pieces of clingfilm and give the thicker ends a bit of a bash with a rolling pin or other heavy object.

3 Now lay out 2 large plates and 1 large bowl. Add the flour and Cajun seasoning to one plate and mix to combine. Crack the egg into the bowl and whisk, and add the breadcrumbs to the remaining plate.

4 Place both chicken breast pieces on to the flour plate, making sure they get a good coating on both sides, then shake off the excess. Dip the pieces into the egg, again ensuring they are well covered before moving on to the breadcrumbs. Carefully toss the chicken in the crumbs, pressing them on to the chicken to get a really good covering.

5 Transfer the breaded chicken pieces to the lined baking tray before carefully drizzling or spraying over the olive oil. Pop them in the oven for 20 minutes, until cooked through, golden and crisp.

6 While they cook, make the coleslaw by adding all the ingredients into a bowl along with a pinch of salt and pepper. Give that a good mix to get everything combined, then leave to one side.

7 To serve, place a baked chicken 'burger' on the bottom of each burger bun, pile on the coleslaw and sliced gherkins, then top with the bun lids. It's a messy one!

veggie quarter-pounder with cheese

*It's easy enough to provide a meaty burger recipe –
but to create a veggie (or even vegan) burger that still has
that depth of flavour, well that's more of a challenge.*

For the burgers

2 tbsp olive oil

80g mushrooms, diced

40g carrots, diced

2 garlic cloves, diced

40g red onion, diced

1 x 400g tin red
  kidney beans,
  drained and rinsed

250g (drained weight)
  cooked Puy lentils,
  drained and rinsed

2 tbsp dark soy sauce

2 tbsp nutritional yeast

1½ tbsp dried
  mixed herbs

75g porridge oats

To serve

6 seeded burger buns

6 cheese slices (such
  as Cheddar)

2 tomatoes, sliced

A couple of handfuls of
  mixed salad leaves

A few gherkins, drained
  and sliced

6 servings of burger
  sauce (see page 233)

1 Preheat the oven to 150°C/130°C fan/Gas Mark 2. Line a baking tray with greaseproof paper.

2 To make the burgers, place a large frying pan over a medium heat and add 1 tablespoon of the oil. Add all the other burger ingredients, except the oats, and pan-fry for 8–10 minutes until softened. Transfer to a food processor along with the oats and blend until all the ingredients are well combined and the mix is the right texture to form into burger patties. Divide and shape the mix into 6 burgers.

3 Get the formed patties on to the lined baking tray and pop in the oven for 10 minutes, then turn over and bake for a further 10 minutes. Remove and leave to cool and firm up.

4 When you are ready to eat, wipe out the frying pan, pop it back over a medium heat and add the remaining tablespoon of oil. Carefully pan-fry the baked burger patties for 3-4 minutes on each side until browned and firm.

5 To serve, split the burger buns (toast them, if you like), add a burger patty to each, then top each with a cheese slice, a couple of tomato slices, a few salad leaves and gherkins. You can pile the tomatoes, leaves, gherkins and burgers into the buns any way you like, but we always like to finish by drizzling over the burger sauce, before adding the bun tops!

Top Tip: Going vegan? If so, remove the cheese slices and use a vegan mayonnaise to make the burger sauce instead, plus make sure your burger buns are vegan too. This will make the meal 490kcal per serving.

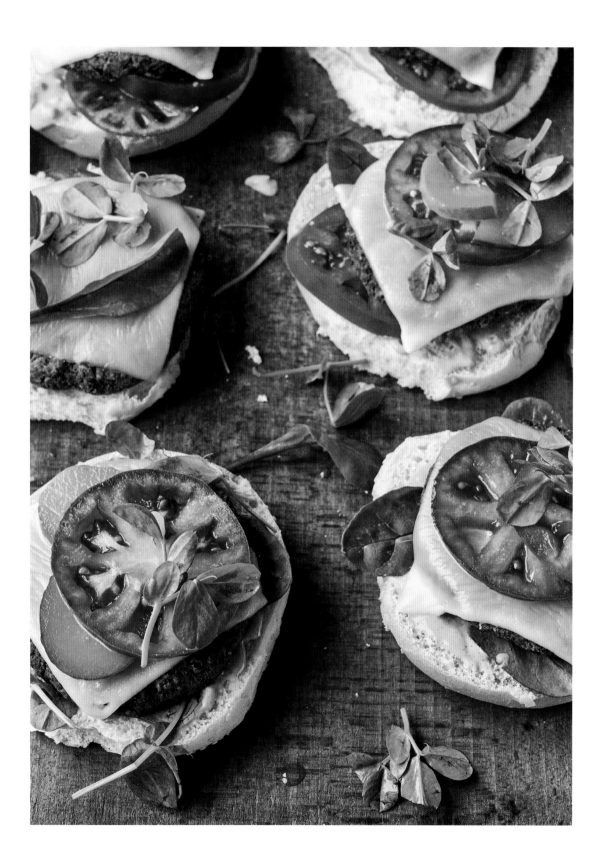

pizza

We love pizza, so there's no way we could live without it as part of a weight loss journey. And there's no reason to, because #itsfine! This is our dough and sauce recipe, and there's an idea for a pizza with toppings in the next recipe.

makes 4 medium bases

500kcal per serving

For the pizza dough

325ml lukewarm water

1½ tsp dried active yeast granules

½ tbsp maple syrup

2 tbsp extra virgin olive oil

500g '00' flour (or strong white bread flour), plus extra for dusting

½ tsp salt

For smaller appetites, make this into 6 bases at 335kcal per serving.

1 For the pizza dough, add the warm water to a jug along with the yeast, maple syrup and olive oil. Give it a whisk and leave for 5 minutes until frothy on top.

2 Next, mix the flour and salt in a bowl and then sift it on to a clean board or work surface (or you can just sift them together and make the dough in the bowl). Make a well in the middle of the flour, then pour the yeasty liquid into the well and carefully stir the flour in. Gradually pull the flour in from the sides into the liquid until it all starts to come together, then get your hands in there and knead the mix until you get a lovely, smooth and elastic dough, about 5–10 minutes.

3 Place the dough in a clean floured bowl and cover with a damp tea towel, then leave to rise in a warm place for around an hour, by which time it should have doubled in size.

4 Transfer the dough on to a floured board or work surface and give it a little knead again, then separate into the number of pizzas you are making and use as required. If you want to freeze it at this stage, double-wrap the dough tightly in clingfilm, either as one batch of dough, or divided into individual portions. When you want to use it, defrost overnight in the fridge, then leave at room temperature for 20 minutes before you shape it.

For the sauce

2 tsp extra virgin olive oil

1 small garlic
clove, minced

270g tinned chopped
tomatoes

40g tomato purée

1 tsp maple syrup

½ tsp dried basil

¼ tsp dried oregano

Salt and ground
black pepper

sauce for
4 medium
pizzas

50kcal
per serving

For smaller
appetites,
make this
into sauces
for 6 pizzas
at 35kcal per
serving.

5 Meanwhile, make the pizza sauce. Place a medium saucepan over a medium heat, add the oil and then the minced garlic. Fry for a couple of minutes, stirring, then add the tomatoes, tomato purée, maple syrup and dried herbs. Add a good pinch of salt and pepper as well. Cover and simmer for 10 minutes, stirring every now and then.

6 Remove the lid and crush up any lumps of tomato until you get a nice, relatively smooth sauce. Let it continue to bubble away, uncovered, until it reaches the consistency you prefer. Use the sauce to top the pizza bases.

7 This sauce (once cooled!) freezes really well, just pop it in a freezerproof tub (or divide into smaller tubs for individual portions) and freeze for up to 6 months, then defrost before use. It will also keep in the fridge for up to 3–4 days.

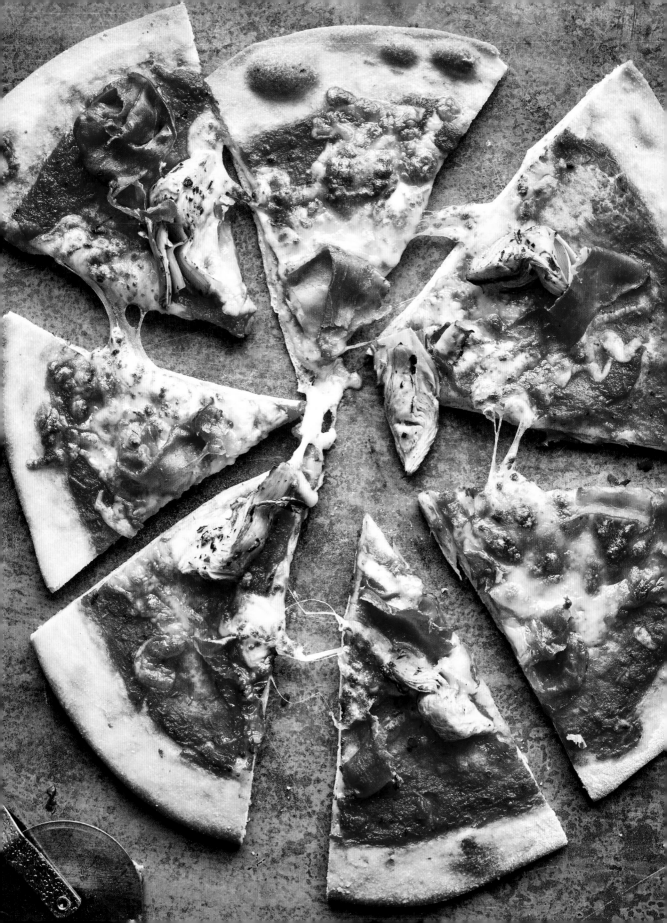

parma ham and artichoke pizza

The great thing about pizzas is you can always customise them to make your own favourite. We've gone for a really simple but completely delicious option here. Less is more when it comes to toppings, so if you do go with your own combination, don't overload it and you won't get the dreaded soggy bottom.

makes 1

730kcal per serving for larger appetites

490kcal per serving for smaller appetites

For larger appetites

1 medium pizza base dough (page 186), plus plain flour for dusting

3 tbsp pizza sauce (page 187)

1½ slices of Parma ham, roughly torn

25g artichoke antipasti, drained

25g mozzarella cheese, thinly sliced

1 tsp olive oil

A few basil leaves

For smaller appetites

1 small pizza base dough (page 186), plus plain flour for dusting

2 tbsp pizza sauce (page 187)

1 slice of Parma ham, roughly torn

15g artichoke antipasti, drained

20g mozzarella cheese, thinly sliced

½ tsp olive oil

A few basil leaves

1 Preheat the oven as high as it will go and pop in a large baking tray.

2 Make sure the pizza dough is at room temperature to make it easier to work with. On a lightly floured board, roll the dough out until you get it down to around ½cm thick. Take your time over this, rotating the dough so you get a nice even base.

3 Place the pizza base on a sheet of greaseproof paper, then spoon on the pizza sauce and carefully spread it out across the base. Drape the pieces of Parma ham around the pizza and chop up the artichokes into smaller bits, scattering those over the base as well. Cover with the mozzarella slices.

4 Carefully remove the baking tray from the oven and transfer the pizza (still on the greaseproof paper) on to it. You may find it easier to turn the baking tray upside down for this. Drizzle the oil around the edge of the pizza crust and then pop it in the oven. Depending on how hot your oven gets, it should take around 8-10 minutes, but keep an eye on it. No one wants burnt pizza!

5 When the pizza is lovely and golden, remove from the oven, scatter over a few torn basil leaves and serve.

the #itsfine chicken tikka masala

The ultimate British curry. Possibly even the ultimate British takeaway! And it's one of those classic meals that's almost easier to make yourself than it is to drive to the restaurant and back. This recipe really can be on your table in under 30 minutes and at a fraction of the cost of eating out.

1 tbsp vegetable oil

450g boneless, skinless chicken breasts, cut into 2–3cm chunks

1 small red onion, finely diced

2 tbsp tomato purée

2 garlic cloves, grated

½ tbsp peeled and grated fresh root ginger

1 tsp garam masala

1 tsp ground turmeric

½ tsp chilli powder (or more to taste)

1 x 400g tin chopped tomatoes

½ chicken stock cube

100ml double cream

200g basmati rice

A small handful of coriander, roughly chopped

Salt and ground black pepper

For smaller appetites, turn this into 4 servings at 490kcal per serving.

1 Place a wok or large frying pan over a medium heat and, when hot, add the oil. Carefully add the chicken chunks to the pan along with the onion, then season with a pinch of salt and pepper and fry for 4-5 minutes, turning regularly.

2 Next up, add the tomato purée, garlic, ginger and the spices. Stir well so everything gets coated, then fry for another couple of minutes before adding in the chopped tomatoes, 150ml of water and the crumbled stock cube. Reduce the heat to low-medium and leave to bubble away and reduce for 10–15 minutes, stirring every now and then. For the last few minutes, add the cream and stir well to combine.

3 While that cooks, pour the dry rice into a cup (or mug) where the rice pretty much fills it. Add the rice to a saucepan along with, using the same cup to measure, twice the amount of boiling water, plus a little splash extra. Place the pan over a medium heat, season with a pinch of salt, then cover and leave to simmer for around 10 minutes until tender. If it gets a little too dry, add a splash more water. When the rice is cooked, drain it, then pour over a little more boiling water, letting that drain off as well. Leave to steam-dry for 5 minutes.

4 Serve up the lovely fluffy white rice, spoon over the chicken and sauce and finish with the coriander sprinkled over. This one is a real winner!

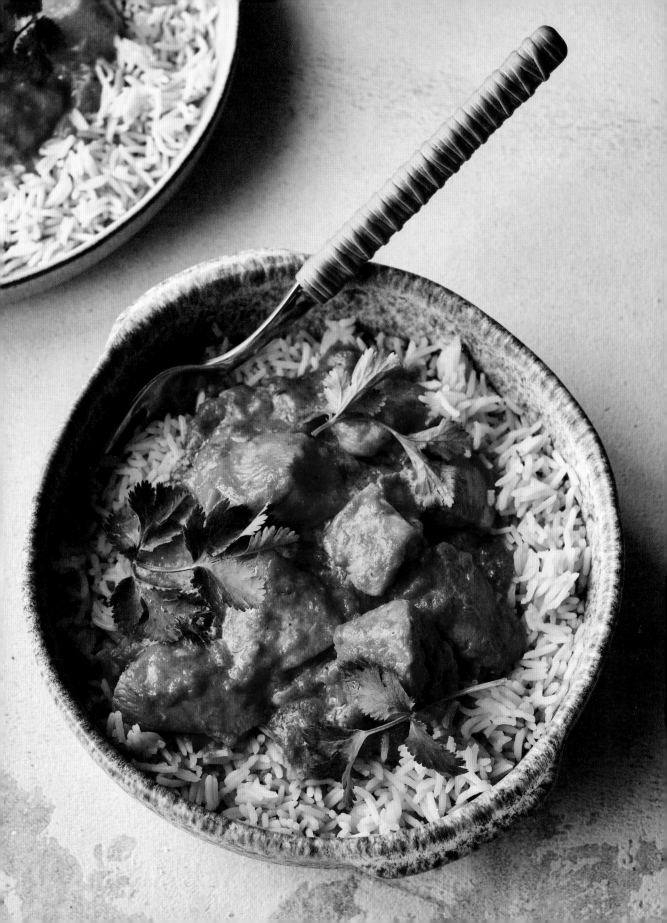

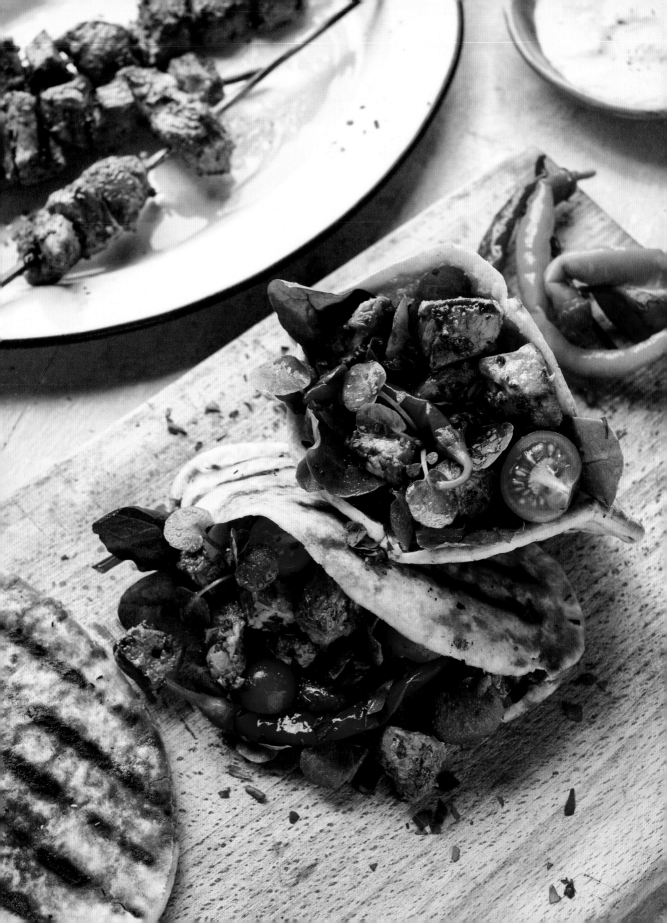

greek-style lamb kebabs

serves 3

485kcal
per serving

Forget your greasy, late-night kebabs. These are a more refined version, made with chunks of lamb instead. Get your lamb pieces marinating two hours in advance, or ideally overnight, as those flavours will really soak into the meat and will transport you away to the Mediterranean.

For the lamb

400g lamb leg steaks, most of the fat removed

Grated zest and juice of 1 lemon

2 garlic cloves, grated

1 tbsp dried oregano

1 tbsp olive oil

Salt and ground black pepper

For the garlic sauce

3 tbsp natural yogurt

2 large garlic cloves, grated

A pinch of salt

To serve

3 pitta breads

2 large handfuls of mixed salad leaves

A handful of parsley, chopped

100g cherry tomatoes, halved

75g pitted black olives, halved

A few pickled chillies, drained (optional)

1 Prepare the lamb. Cut the lamb steaks into bite-sized chunks, around 2cm each, and place into a sandwich bag or container. Add the lemon zest and juice, garlic, oregano and olive oil along with a good pinch of salt and pepper. Give them a good mix up to get all those flavours combined and into the meat, then seal the bag or cover the container and pop in the fridge for at least 2 hours (or ideally overnight) until ready to cook.

2 At that point, get the lamb pieces on to some skewers. Metal skewers are ideal, but if you only have wooden ones, soak them in water for around an hour before using.

3 Get the barbecue nice and hot, or alternatively you can cook them under a preheated hot grill. Pop the skewers over/under the heat and let them cook for 10–15 minutes in total, turning every few minutes. Don't be afraid to get some lovely caramelised bits, as that's all flavour!

4 While they cook, knock up a super simple garlic sauce by mixing the yogurt with the grated garlic and the pinch of salt in a small bowl.

5 To serve, pop the pittas into a warm oven or over the barbecue (or under the grill) for a minute on each side, which will help you to split them open. Now you can just pile the salad leaves, parsley and tomatoes into the warm pittas, top with the lamb and then the olives and chillies (if using). Drizzle over that garlic sauce and bang, you are back on your holidays!

a cheeky piri-piri chicken

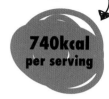

serves 4

740kcal per serving

We all know where you go for your piri-piri fix, but how about not having to leave the house for it?

For the chicken
700g boneless, skinless chicken thighs

Juice of 1 lemon

2 garlic cloves, grated

A few sprigs of thyme

For the rice
2 tsp olive oil

1 small red onion, finely diced

1 tsp ground cumin

1 tsp ground turmeric

½ tsp smoked paprika

A pinch of dried chilli flakes (or to taste)

230g long-grain white rice

1 chicken stock cube

1 roasted red pepper from a jar (or a home-roasted one), drained and diced

For the piri-piri sauce
1 large red chilli, deseeded and finely diced

1 large garlic clove, chopped

A pinch of salt

2 tbsp olive oil

½ tbsp lemon juice

For the peas
350g frozen peas

1 red chilli, deseeded and finely diced

3 tbsp butter

1 tsp finely chopped mint

A handful of coriander, chopped

1 For the chicken, place the chicken thighs in a bowl with the lemon juice, garlic and thyme. Give that a good mix to combine and leave to marinate at room temperature for 15 minutes.

2 Meanwhile, make the rice by placing a frying pan over a medium heat and adding the oil. When hot, add the onion and fry for a few minutes until starting to soften. Add all the spices along with the rice and continue to cook for another minute, making sure you stir the mixture well so the rice gets coated in all the spices.

3 Next up, add 500ml of water along with the crumbled stock cube and the roasted red pepper. Give that a stir, bring to the boil, then drop the heat down to low and cover. Leave that to cook for around 30 minutes, stirring regularly.

4 Back to the chicken now, so get the grill to a medium-high heat and add the chicken thighs to a wire rack set over a baking tray to catch any escaping juices (or use the grill rack and grill pan). Place under the grill and cook for 5 minutes on each side, turning once.

5 Meanwhile, make the piri-piri sauce by adding the chopped chilli and garlic to a pestle and mortar. Add the salt and mix until you get a smooth paste. Add the oil and lemon juice and combine. You can also make this in a small food processor.

6 After 10 minutes, remove the chicken from the grill and cover it with the piri-piri sauce, then place it back under the grill for another 5 minutes on each side.

7 Pop the peas into a pan, add enough boiling water to cover and simmer for around 3-4 minutes. Drain and add back to the saucepan along with the chilli, butter and herbs. Give some of the peas a mash with the back of a fork as you stir it all together.

For smaller appetites, turn this into 6 servings at 495kcal per serving.

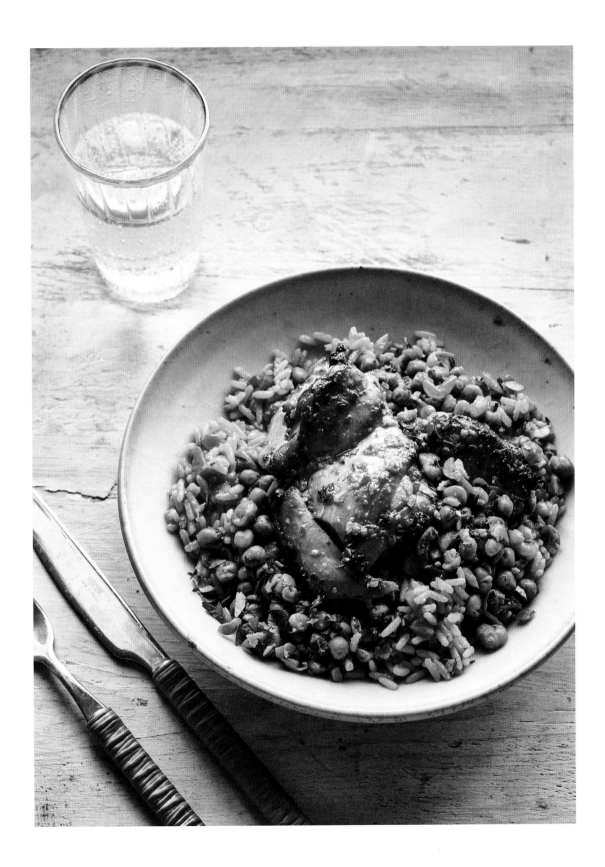

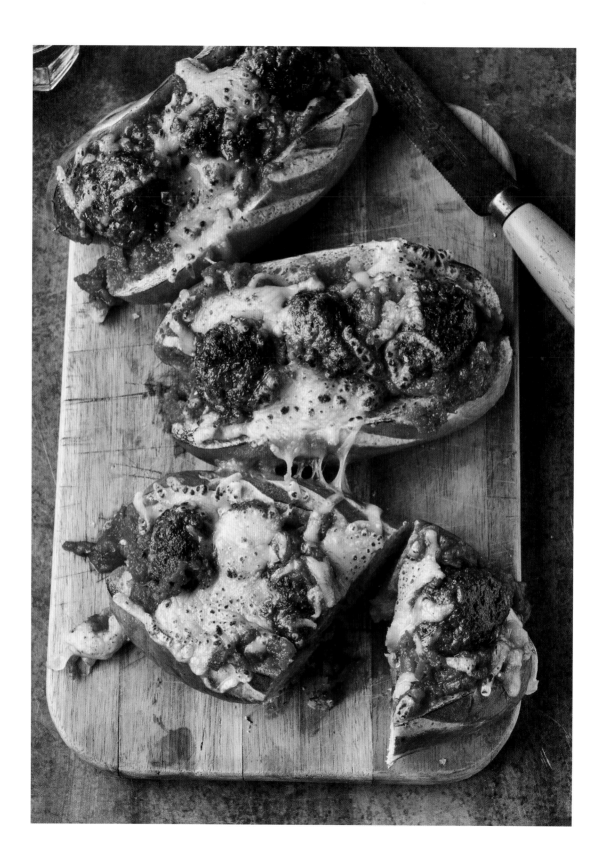

the mighty meatball sub

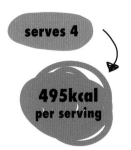

serves 4

495kcal per serving

We do love a good sandwich, and there are a few great options when you visit that famous sub shop. But, without a doubt, our go-to is always the meatball sub. It's a bit of a messy one, and ours is no different — so we would suggest a knife and fork might come in handy!

500g minced beef (5 per cent fat)

1 tbsp dried Italian herb seasoning

1 tsp salt, plus an extra good pinch

1 tsp ground black pepper, plus an extra good pinch

2 tbsp olive oil

1 small garlic clove, minced

1 x 400g tin chopped tomatoes

60g tomato purée

1 tsp maple syrup

½ tsp dried basil

¼ tsp dried oregano

4 hot-dog buns

80g mozzarella cheese, grated

1 Preheat the oven to 170°C/150°C fan/Gas Mark 3½.

2 Add the minced beef to a large bowl along with the Italian herb seasoning and the teaspoon each of salt and pepper. Give the meat a good squish and squeeze, so that you get all those flavours mixed all the way through, then form into around 12 ping pong ball-sized meatballs.

3 Pop a large frying pan over a medium heat and add half of the olive oil. When hot, carefully add the meatballs and fry for 10–15 minutes, turning regularly, until browned on all sides.

4 While they cook, in a medium saucepan over a medium heat, add the remaining oil and the garlic. Fry for a couple of minutes, stirring, then add the tomatoes, tomato purée, maple syrup and herbs. Add a good pinch of salt and pepper as well. Cover and simmer for 10 minutes, stirring every now and then.

5 Remove the lid and crush up any lumps of tomato until you get a nice, relatively smooth sauce. Let it continue to bubble away, uncovered, until it reaches the consistency you prefer.

6 Split open all of the hot-dog buns, but try to keep them each as one piece. Flatten them out as best you can, place on a nonstick baking tray and add 3 meatballs to each. Cover with the sauce, share out the mozzarella over the top of each one and then bake for 5–10 minutes, until the cheese is all gooey and golden.

hong kong-style sweet and sour chicken

serves 4

670kcal per serving

An absolute takeaway classic here, but done the #itsfine way. Sweet, sticky and completely delicious, we think this one will become a firm favourite in your house.

2 tbsp cornflour

2 medium eggs, beaten

80g plain flour

2 tsp sweet paprika

700g boneless, skinless chicken breasts, cut into bite-sized pieces

60ml vegetable oil

1 white onion, cut into bite-sized pieces

1 green pepper, deseeded and cut into bite-sized pieces

1 red pepper, deseeded and cut into bite-sized pieces

2 garlic cloves, minced

1 thumb-sized piece of fresh root ginger, peeled and minced

130ml passata

20ml red wine vinegar

60g light soft brown sugar

230g tinned pineapple chunks in juice (with the juice)

160g long-grain white rice

2 spring onions, chopped

Salt and ground black pepper

1 Get yourself 3 bowls out, add the cornflour to one, the beaten eggs to another and finally the flour, paprika and a good pinch of salt and pepper, well mixed, to the final bowl. Toss the chicken chunks in the cornflour, then shake off the excess from each piece and transfer to the egg. Make sure each piece is fully coated, then move them into the seasoned flour. Toss them through again to get a good coating.

2 Next up, add 40ml of the oil to a large frying pan over a medium-high heat. Add the chicken and cook, turning regularly, until golden brown, for around 5–8 minutes. Don't overcrowd the pan, so you may need to do this in 2 batches. When they are all cooked, transfer to a plate and leave to one side.

3 Give the pan a wipe with some kitchen paper, place back over a medium-high heat and add the remaining oil. Add the onion and peppers and stir-fry for a few minutes, then add the garlic and ginger. Continue to cook for 1–2 minutes before adding the passata, vinegar, sugar and the pineapple chunks and juice. Get that simmering away and leave to bubble, uncovered, for 5–10 minutes until lovely and thick. Add the chicken back in, stir well to coat it in the sauce, then cook for 5 minutes to get it all piping hot.

4 While the chicken mix cooks, cook the rice in a pan of lightly salted boiling water, according to the packet instructions. When it's ready, drain, then serve topped with the sweet and sour chicken and finish with the spring onions.

For smaller appetites, turn this into 6 servings at 445kcal per serving.

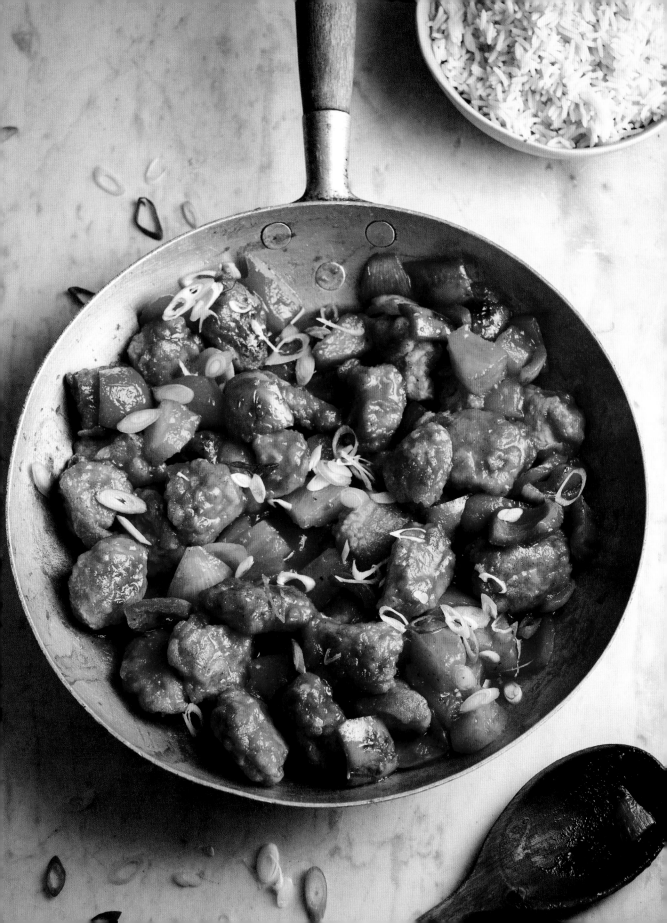

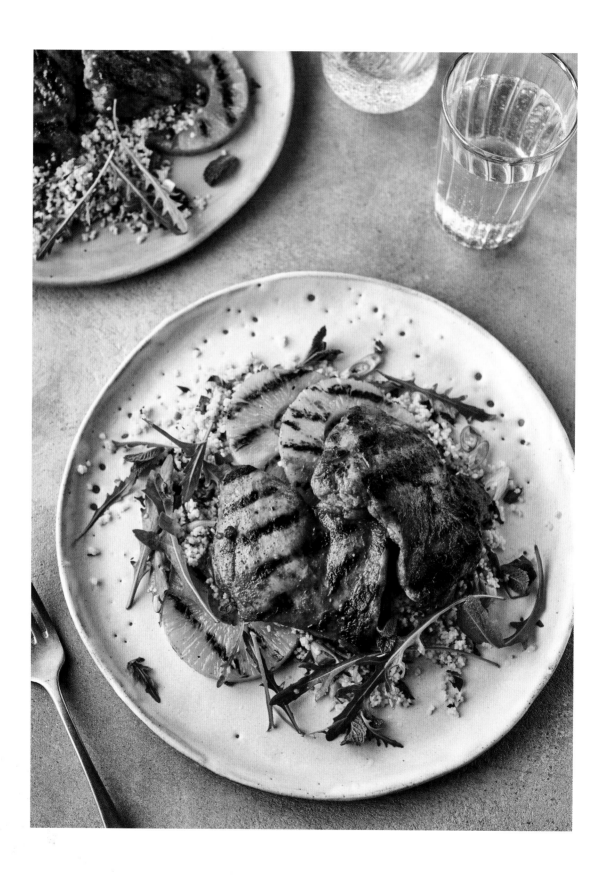

this chicken ain't no jerk

This isn't jerk chicken, but it's certainly inspired by it. It's tamer in the spice department, but the pineapple in the marinade and the couscous makes this something really special.

1 x 425g tin pineapple rings in juice

1 tsp cayenne pepper

¼ tsp garlic granules

¼ tsp ground ginger

½ tsp onion granules

A pinch of ground allspice

1 tsp za'atar (or dried thyme)

1½ tbsp light soy sauce

4 boneless, skinless chicken thighs

Vegetable oil, for brushing

100g couscous

Boiling water, to cover

A small handful of mint leaves, finely chopped

A handful of parsley, finely chopped

2 spring onions, finely chopped

A few handfuls of rocket leaves

Salt and ground black pepper

For smaller appetites, turn this into 3 servings at 430kcal per serving.

1 Start by separating the pineapple from the juice. Keep the rings to one side, then take 2 tablespoons of the juice and add to a large bowl along with the spices and soy sauce. Give that a whisk, then add the chicken thighs, making sure they get a good mix to get a lovely coating all over them. Leave to marinate for at least an hour, or even overnight, in the fridge.

2 To cook the chicken, it's best done over a hot barbecue, brushing the grill rack with oil first. They will take around 15 minutes, turning every few minutes. Or you can pop them under a preheated hot grill for around 20 minutes in total, flipping a few times as they cook.

3 With about 5 minutes to go, place the pineapple rings over the barbecue or under the grill alongside the chicken and cook, turning halfway through, so they get some nice char marks on them.

4 While the chicken cooks, place the couscous in a heatproof bowl and pour over some boiling water, adding enough water to cover the couscous plus a couple more tablespoons. Place a tea towel (or clingfilm) over the bowl and leave for 5 minutes, by which time the water should have been absorbed, then give the soft grains a good fluff up with a fork. Add the chopped herbs and spring onions and another 2-3 tablespoons of pineapple juice along with a good pinch of salt and pepper. Stir well to combine.

5 To serve, pile the couscous on to serving plates, top with the chicken and charred pineapple rings and serve the rocket on the side.

chinese pork belly tacos

This dish takes two of our favourite cuisines, Mexican and Chinese, and mixes them together into something a little bit special.

For the pork

500g pork belly slices

1 chicken stock cube

3 garlic cloves (2 roughly chopped, 1 grated)

1½ tbsp runny honey

1 tbsp peeled and grated fresh root ginger

2 tbsp rice wine vinegar

½ tbsp light soy sauce

½ red chilli, deseeded and finely diced

1 tbsp vegetable oil

For the slaw

100g carrots, grated

60g white or red cabbage, thinly sliced

2 large spring onions, finely sliced

1 red pepper, deseeded and thinly sliced

A large handful of coriander, chopped

1½ tbsp extra virgin olive oil

½ tbsp peeled and grated fresh root ginger

1 garlic clove, grated

½ tbsp light soy sauce

1 tbsp rice wine vinegar

½ tbsp sesame oil

½ tbsp runny honey

8 small tortillas, to serve

1 For the pork, place a large saucepan over a medium heat and add 500ml of water. Add the pork belly slices, crumbled stock cube, the 2 chopped garlic cloves, ½ tablespoon of the honey, half of the ginger and ½ tablespoon of the vinegar. Bring to the boil, then drop to a gentle simmer and cover, leaving it to bubble away for around 1½ hours. Remove the pork belly slices and leave to one side. Discard the rest.

2 Grab a bowl and add the grated garlic clove, the remaining honey, ginger and vinegar, the soy sauce, chilli and half the vegetable oil. Mix well to combine.

3 Place a large wok or frying pan over a high heat and add the remaining veg oil. Cut the pork into 2.5cm pieces and, when the oil is nice and hot, carefully add the pork and stir-fry for a couple of minutes before adding in the sauce. Continue to fry for a few minutes, turning the pork regularly in the sticky glaze.

4 While the pork cooks, knock the slaw up quickly by adding the prepped vegetables and coriander to a large bowl. In a small bowl, mix together all the remaining ingredients and then pour over the veggies. Toss well to make sure everything gets coated.

5 To serve, wrap the tortillas in foil and warm in a preheated oven (around 160°C/140°C fan/Gas Mark 3) for 5 minutes, then pile some slaw into each one and top with the sweet and sticky pork pieces. Get stuck in!

> **For smaller appetites, turn this into 6 servings at 480kcal per serving.**

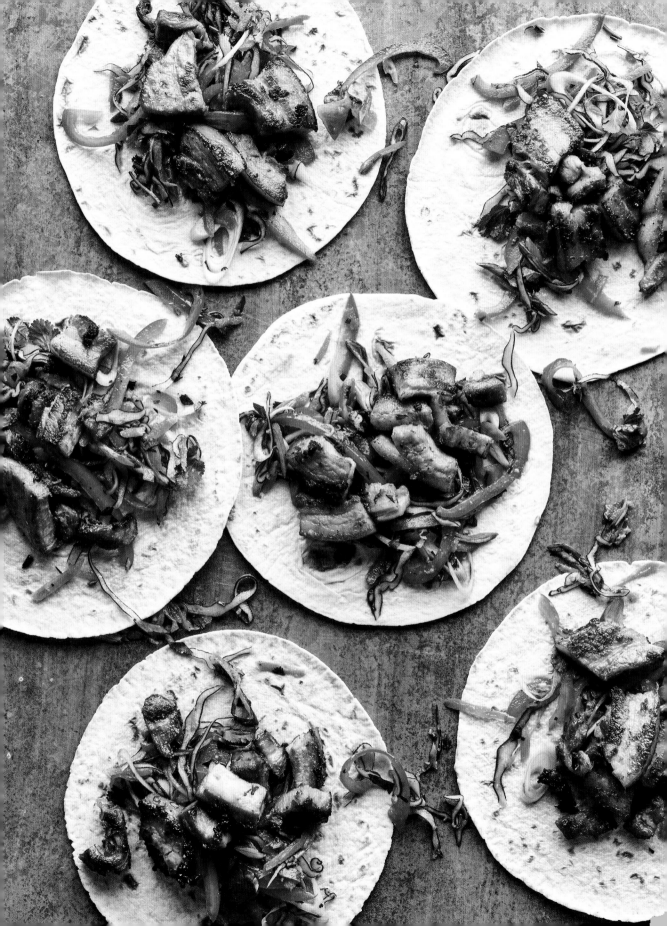

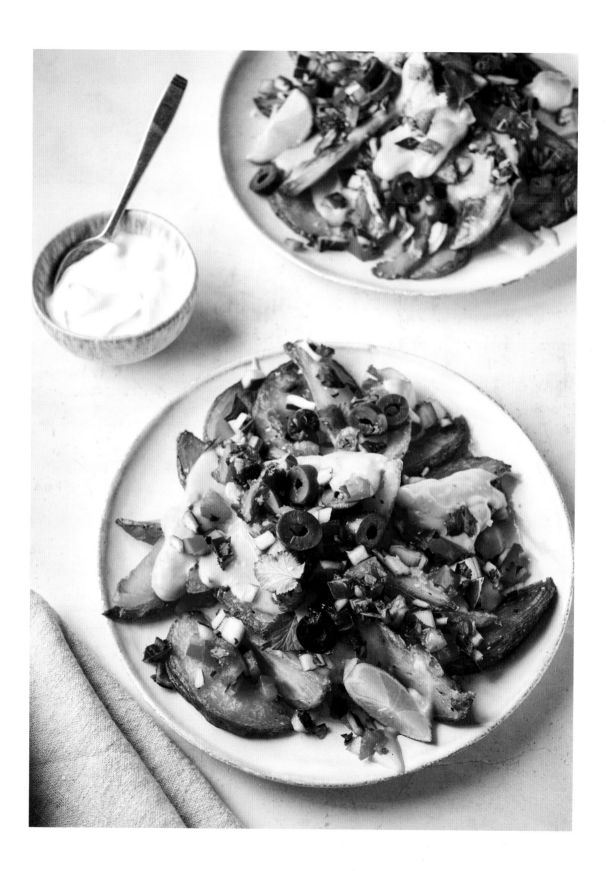

'nacho' average nachos

We all know what nachos are like, don't we? They are pretty darn tasty and a great choice when going to your favourite Tex-Mex restaurant. But we wanted to do something a bit different, and we came up with these. We're not saying they are better, but we're not saying they aren't either!

For the potato 'nachos'

800g white potatoes, cut into thin wedges

1 tbsp vegetable oil

Salt and ground black pepper

For the salsa

½ red onion, finely diced

1 jalapeño chilli, finely diced (and deseeded if preferred)

A pinch of salt

Juice of ½ lime

1 large tomato, finely diced

A small bunch of coriander, chopped, plus extra to garnish

For the nacho cheese sauce

1 tbsp butter

1 tbsp plain flour

150ml semi-skimmed milk

65g spicy Cheddar cheese, grated

To garnish

40g pitted black olives, sliced

2 tbsp soured cream

1 Preheat the oven to 170°C/150°C fan/Gas Mark 3½.

2 For the potato nachos, pop the potato wedges into a pan of boiling water and cook for 5 minutes, then drain and leave to steam-dry for another 5 minutes. Place on a baking tray, pour over the oil and season with a good couple of pinches of salt and pepper. Toss the wedges around to make sure everything gets coated, then spread them out on the baking tray. Bake for 35-40 minutes, turning at least once, until golden and crisp.

3 Meanwhile, for the salsa, just add the onion and chilli to a bowl along with the salt and lime juice. Give it a good mix and let that sit for about 5 minutes, before stirring through the tomato and chopped coriander. Leave to one side.

4 Next up, make the nacho cheese sauce by gently melting the butter in a small saucepan, then add the flour and whisk well to incorporate, letting the mix cook out for a minute. Add the milk in batches, adding a small amount at the start, then gradually adding more and more, whisking as you go to get rid of any lumps. When all the milk is incorporated, add the grated Cheddar and stir that through.

5 Now it's just a case of assembling the dish by adding the cooked wedges to a large serving plate or tray. Pour over the nacho cheese sauce and then top with the salsa. Garnish with the olives, dollops of soured cream and some more chopped coriander.

Top Tip: If you don't fancy the spicy Cheddar, just replace it with the same amount of standard Cheddar.

For smaller appetites, turn this into 3 servings at 500kcal per serving.

wham, bam, thank you lamb

Typically this would be a goat curry, but this version with diced lamb still tastes pretty authentic. It's a hot one, so adjust that Scotch bonnet or remove it if you want to make it less spicy.

For the curry

1 tbsp vegetable oil

600g diced lamb (lean)

4 garlic cloves, minced

2 tsp peeled and minced fresh root ginger

2 large white onions, diced

1 spring onion, finely diced

½ Scotch bonnet chilli (or to taste), finely diced

2 tsp Madras curry powder

A couple of sprigs of thyme, leaves picked

1 tbsp tomato purée

200g white potatoes, diced

For the rice and beans

200g long-grain white rice

400ml light coconut milk

1 x 400g tin red kidney beans, drained and rinsed

½ Scotch bonnet chilli (or to taste), finely diced

2 spring onions, finely diced

A sprig of thyme, leaves picked

Salt

1 Start with the curry. Place a saucepan over a medium heat and when hot, add the oil, then fry the lamb until browned all over, about 5-10 minutes. You may need to do this in batches depending on how big your pan is.

2 When all the meat is browned and back in the pan, add in the garlic, ginger, onions, spring onion and Scotch bonnet chilli along with the curry powder, thyme leaves and tomato purée. Stir well, top up with enough water to just cover the meat, then leave to simmer for an hour or until the lamb is tender, adding water as required if it gets too dry. Add the diced potato for the last 15 minutes.

3 Towards the end of the curry cooking time, make the rice and beans. Add the rice to a separate pan of salted boiling water and simmer for 10 minutes until tender.

4 Drain the rice, then add it back into the pan along with the coconut milk, kidney beans, Scotch bonnet chilli, spring onions and thyme leaves. Stir well and allow it to heat through for a few minutes, before serving with the lamb curry.

Top Tip: Scotch bonnet chillies are very hot, so if you want to make this a little cooler, remove the seeds. You could also swap it with a standard red chilli, or even remove it altogether. Whichever chilli you use though, we would recommend wearing latex gloves when you chop it.

For smaller appetites, turn this into 6 servings at 430kcal per serving.

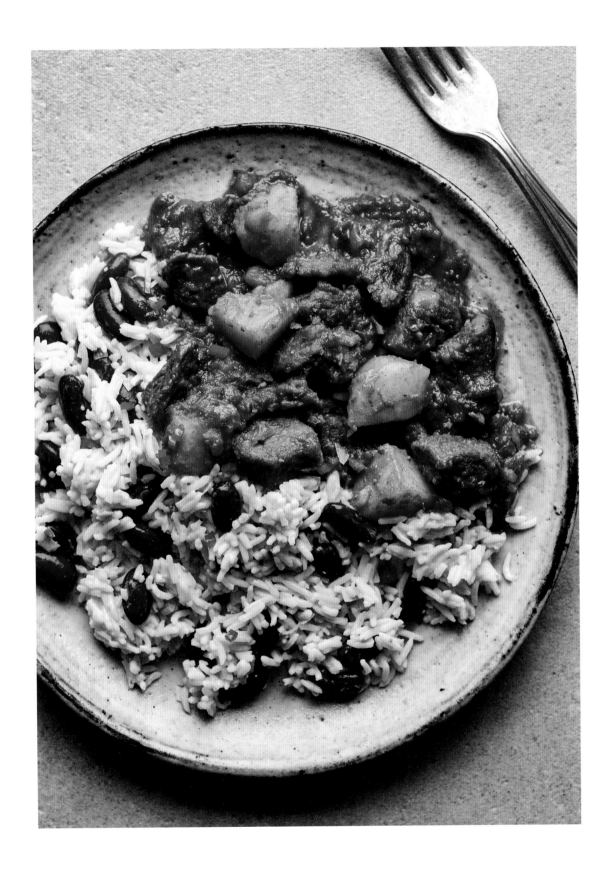

banging bites

gnocchi pops

serves 4

270kcal
per serving

We are big fans of gnocchi at #itsfine HQ. But it doesn't always have to be part of a main course, you can also turn it into these delicious little bites. Crisp on the outside and chewy on the inside, they really are the perfect snack.

1 x 500g packet
  long-life gnocchi
1 tbsp olive oil
1½ tsp smoked paprika
100g natural yogurt
1 tsp harissa paste
Salt

1 Preheat the oven to 170°C/150°C fan/Gas Mark 3½. Line a baking tray with greaseproof paper.

2 Carefully add the gnocchi to a large pan of lightly salted boiling water. Let them bubble away for just a minute, then drain. Lay the gnocchi out on a tray or a plate and leave them to steam-dry for a few minutes.

3 Add the gnocchi to a bowl and toss in the oil and paprika, making sure every piece gets a coating. Place on the lined baking tray in a single layer, then pop in the oven for 20–25 minutes, or until lovely and golden, giving them a turn halfway through.

4 While they cook, add the yogurt to a small bowl and spoon in the harissa. Give it a good swirl to mix the two together.

5 Now it's just a case of taking the gnocchi pops from the oven and serving them up with the harissa yogurt.

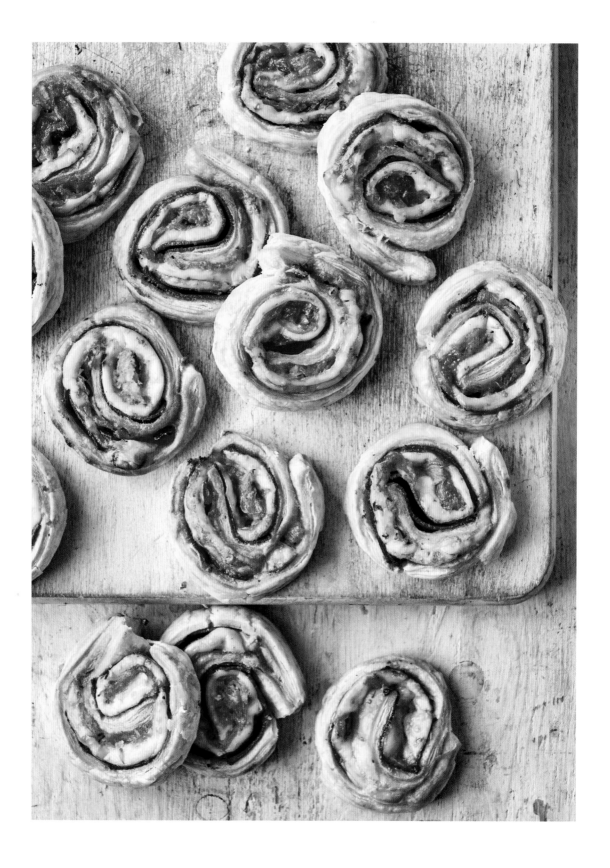

reuben rollups

makes 14

175kcal per serving

Some people may think it's wrong to muck around with a Reuben sandwich, after all, it is a deli classic. But we don't think that way, and using your imagination with the Reuben's ingredients, you can come up with something pretty amazing.

30g mayonnaise (page 231)

30g tomato ketchup

1 tsp hot sauce

1 tsp Worcestershire sauce

3 gherkins, drained and finely diced

¼ tsp smoked paprika

1 x 320g packet chilled fresh ready-rolled puff pastry sheet

10 slices of pastrami

150g Emmental cheese, thinly sliced

120g sauerkraut

A little semi-skimmed milk, for brushing

1 Preheat the oven to 180°C/160°C fan/Gas Mark 4. Line a large baking tray with greaseproof paper (see step 5).

2 First off, get the sauce together by adding the mayonnaise, tomato ketchup, hot sauce, Worcestershire sauce, gherkins and paprika to a small bowl. Give them a good mix to get everything combined, then set to one side.

3 Unroll the pastry sheet on a board or work surface and then lay the slices of pastrami down the length of the pastry sheet – you should be able to cover around two-thirds of the sheet. Top with the cheese and sauerkraut before drizzling over the sauce.

4 Carefully roll the pastry up, starting with the filling side from a long edge. Try and keep it as tight as you can, then when you have almost rolled it all up, brush the final part of the pastry with a little milk to help it stick together and roll it up completely.

5 Using a sharp knife, cut across the pastry roll into even slices, aiming for 14 individual portions. Place them flat (cut side down) on the lined baking tray and pop in the oven for around 20 minutes, until the pastry is lovely and golden and crisp. Depending on the size of your oven and baking tray, you may need to bake them in a couple of batches as they will puff up and spread out a little, so give them a few centimetres space in between each slice.

6 Remove from the oven and serve warm. Store any cold leftovers in the fridge for up to 3-4 days.

mango hot sauce chicken wings

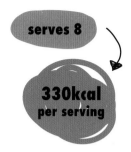

A good chicken wing is something that should be celebrated. And we all know that the sauce is the most important part. Well, these wings are no different, and this sauce is the perfect blend of sweet and spicy.

1kg chicken wings
2 tbsp Cajun seasoning
200g frozen mango chunks
2 tbsp hot sauce
2 tbsp runny honey
30g butter

1 Preheat the oven to 180°C/160°C fan/Gas Mark 4.

2 Add the chicken wings to a large bowl and sprinkle over the Cajun seasoning. Give everything a good mix and massage to get all those flavours into the chicken, then place in a single layer on a wire rack set over a baking tray and roast in the oven for 35 minutes.

3 While they cook, add the mango to a food processor and blitz well until you get a powder. Add that to a large frying pan along with the hot sauce, honey and butter, plus a tablespoon of water. Heat the mix gently for about 5 minutes, stirring regularly, until you get a lovely thick sauce, perfect for coating the wings.

4 After 35 minutes of roasting, remove the wings from the oven and add them in batches to the mango sauce. Make sure you get a good covering over each wing, then pop them back on the wire rack over the baking tray and into the oven for a final 5-10 minutes.

5 When the wings are lovely and sticky, with those perfect crispy bits starting to show, then they are ready to eat.

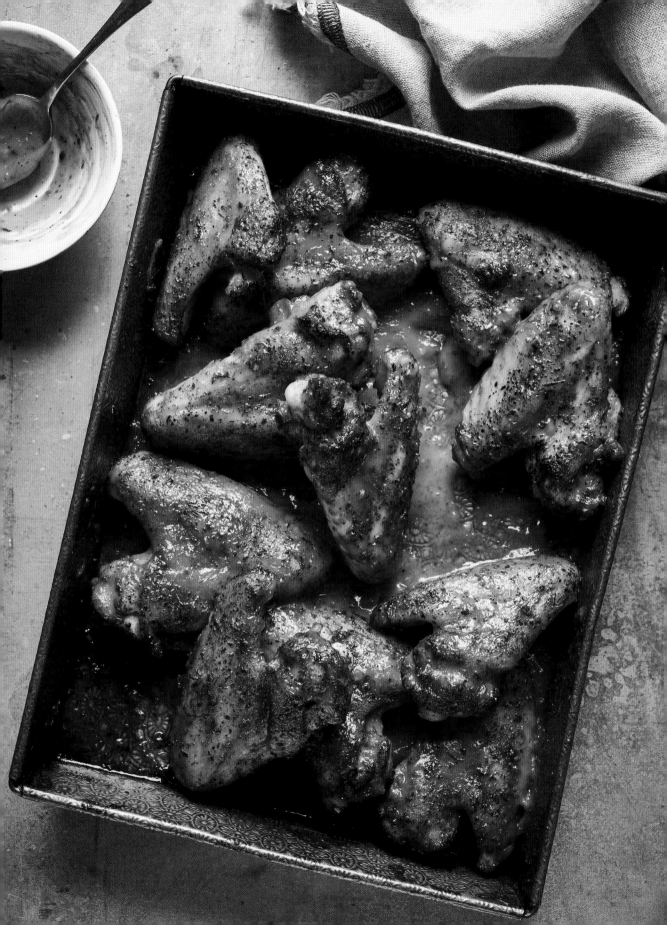

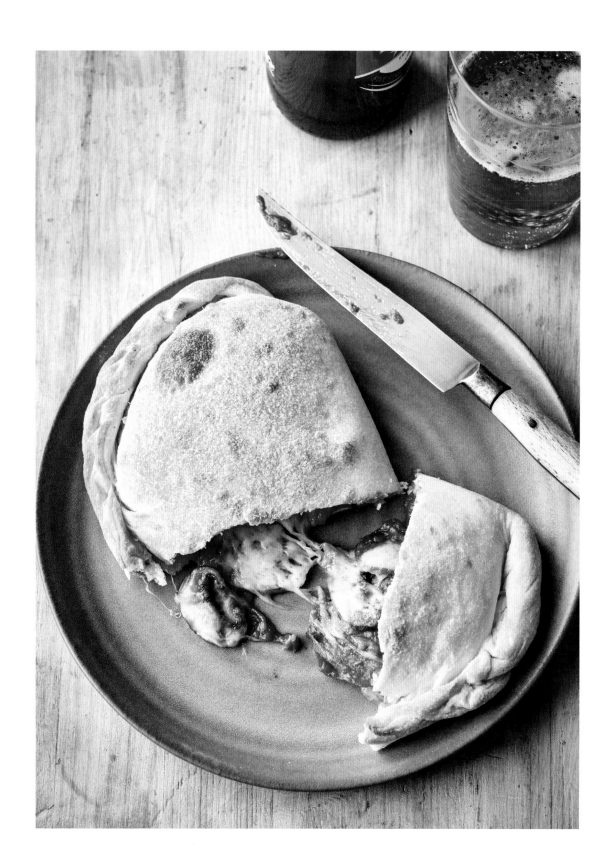

pizza pockets

serves 1

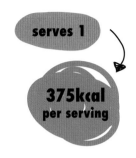

375kcal per serving

Think Cornish pasty, but it's a pizza inside!
Use the pizza dough and pizza sauce recipes from
page 186, which are enough to make 8 pizza pockets.

Plain flour, for dusting

1 serving of pizza dough (page 186)

1 serving of pizza sauce (around 1½ tbsp) (page 187)

2 slices of pepperoni

1 chestnut mushroom, sliced

20g mozzarella cheese, sliced

Olive oil, for brushing

1 Preheat the oven as high as it will go and pop in a baking tray.

2 On a lightly floured board or work surface, roll the dough out into a rough circle, around ½cm thick. Add the pizza sauce into the middle and pile all the other ingredients on top. Carefully fold the dough over to enclose the filling, making sure nothing is poking out of the sides. Crimp the edges by pinching them together between 2 fingers and then fold over. Repeat all the way around the pizza pocket.

3 Place on a piece of greaseproof paper and brush with a tiny bit of oil, then carefully place on the hot baking tray and bake for around 8 minutes or until lovely and golden.

4 Remove from the oven and let it cool slightly before tucking in (as the filling will be very hot!).

arancini with mushroom sauce

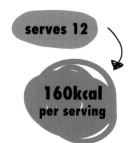

serves 12

160kcal per serving

Arancini are little breaded balls of risotto goodness. They are packed with Parmesan, baked and served up with this awesome mushroom sauce.

For 12 arancini

1 litre boiling water

2 vegetable stock cubes

10g butter

1 red onion, finely diced

2 garlic cloves,
  finely diced

A few sprigs of thyme,
  leaves picked

150g risotto rice

40g Parmesan cheese,
  finely grated

30g plain flour

70g panko breadcrumbs

1 large egg

Salt and ground
  black pepper

For 12 servings of sauce

10g butter

½ small red onion,
  finely diced

1 large garlic clove,
  finely diced

150g mushrooms, sliced

A few sprigs of thyme,
  leaves picked

100ml white wine

150ml chicken stock

100ml double cream

¼ tsp cornflour

1 Start by making the risotto for the arancini. Add the boiling water to a large saucepan, then crumble in the stock cubes. Keep the stock over a low heat while you place a large, high-sided frying pan over a medium heat. Add the butter and then the onion and fry gently for around 5 minutes until starting to soften. Add the garlic and thyme leaves along with a good pinch of salt and pepper. Continue to cook for another 2-3 minutes.

2 Add the rice and stir well, frying for 1-2 minutes more. Now start to add the hot stock, 2 ladlefuls at a time. Make sure the liquid is absorbed each time before you add the next lot. Stir regularly to get a creamy texture. It should take around 20-25 minutes in total.

3 When almost all the stock is added, taste the rice to see if it's cooked. There should be no nuttiness left and the rice should be quite soft. Stir in the Parmesan, then remove from the heat and season to taste. Transfer to a heatproof bowl and leave to cool for 30 minutes, then pop in the fridge to chill for a good 2-3 hours.

4 When making the arancini, preheat the oven to 170°C/150°C fan/ Gas Mark 3½. Line a baking tray with greaseproof paper.

5 Get 2 plates and 1 large bowl out. Put the flour on one plate with a pinch of salt and pepper, the breadcrumbs on another and crack the egg into the bowl and whisk.

6 Wet your hands a little, then divide and roll the risotto into 12 compact golf ball-sized portions. One by one, roll them in the flour to coat, then dip them into the egg to make sure they are completely coated. Finally, pop them into the breadcrumbs and roll them around again for a nice covering. Place on the lined baking tray and pop in the oven for 20 minutes until crisp and golden.

7 While they cook, you can make the sauce. Place a frying pan over a medium heat and melt the butter. Add the onion and fry for 5 minutes to soften, then add the garlic, mushrooms and thyme leaves. Continue to fry for another 5 minutes to get the mushrooms nice and soft, then add the wine. Crank up the heat and let that cook until the wine has almost all been absorbed, then drop the heat back to medium and add the stock and cream.

8 Leave that to simmer gently for 5–10 minutes, until reduced by half. Mix the cornflour with ½ teaspoon of water in a small bowl and add to the sauce. Stir well as it thickens, then remove from the heat.

9 Serve up the arancini either with the sauce on the side, or poured over the top. Totally delicious.

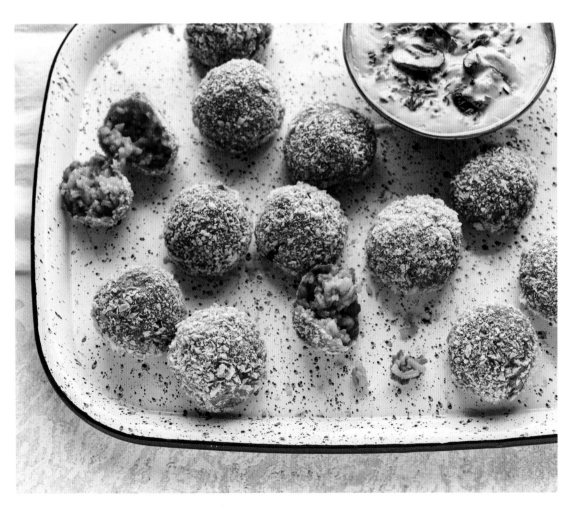

stuffed french toast rollers

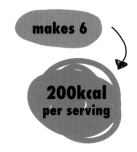

Here we have a lovely savoury version of French toast. Trust us, this recipe really is lovely! These rollers are stuffed with mushrooms, spinach and cheese . . . have we won you over now?

2 tsp butter, plus 1 tbsp

120g mushrooms, finely diced

A few sprigs of thyme, leaves picked

100g fresh spinach

80g Cheddar cheese, grated

6 slices of white bread

½ tsp plain flour

1 medium egg

2 tbsp semi-skimmed milk

Salt and ground black pepper

1 Place a large frying pan over a medium heat and melt the 2 teaspoons of butter. Add the mushrooms and thyme leaves along with a good pinch of salt and pepper. Let those cook away for 5 minutes to get lovely and soft, then add the spinach and let that wilt down, stirring regularly – this should only take a couple of minutes. Adjust the seasoning to taste, then tip the mix into a heatproof bowl and leave to cool for 15–20 minutes. Stir in the cheese.

2 Carefully remove the crusts from the bread, then roll out each slice so they all get quite flat and thinner. Mix the flour in a small bowl with the same quantity of water. Share the mushroom mix out across each slice, piling it up at one end and leaving a gap on either side. Roll each slice up to make a tube stuffed with the filling. Using your finger, wet the edges of the bread with the flour mix to help them stick together. Pinch the ends together to seal them, repeating this for all the slices.

3 Heat the remaining 1 tablespoon of butter in a large frying pan over a medium heat until melted. Meanwhile, in a large bowl, mix together the egg and milk along with a pinch of salt and pepper. Add half of the rollers into the egg/milk mix and let them get a good soaking, rolling them around so everything gets coated.

4 Transfer to the pan and cook for 2–3 minutes on each side, so they get a lovely colour. Transfer to a plate and keep warm while you repeat this with the remaining rollers. Serve hot.

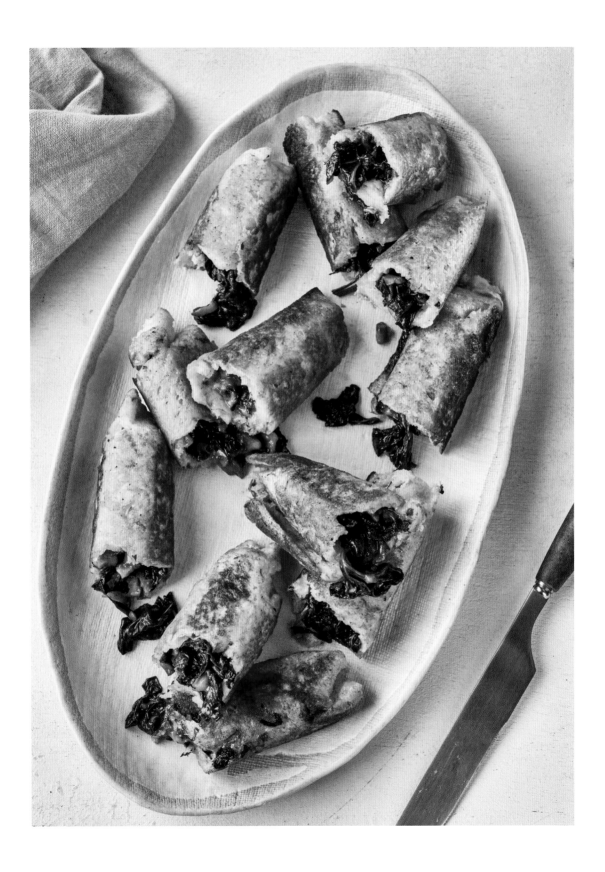

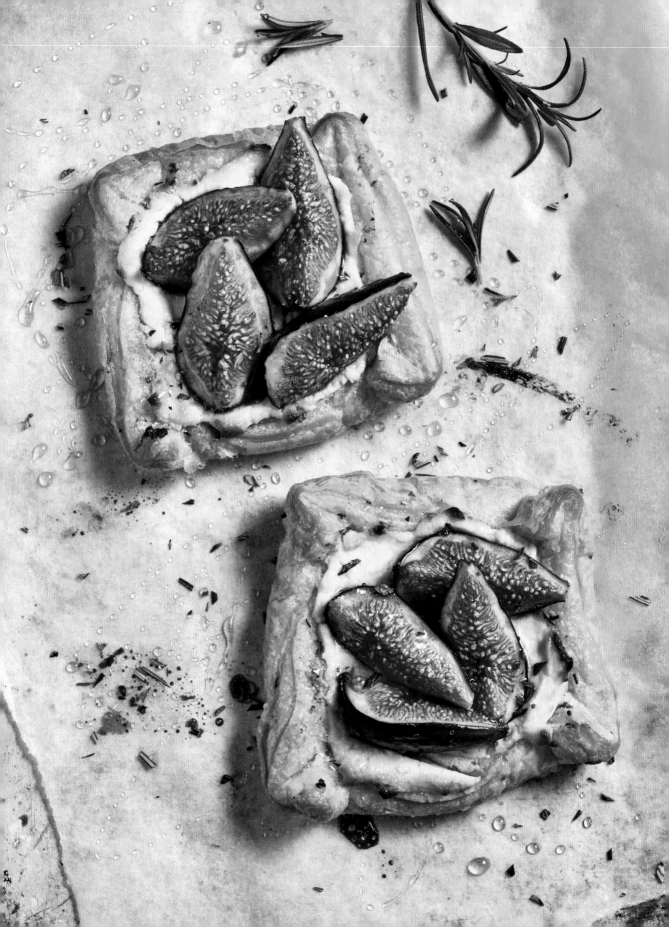

goats' cheese, fig and honey puffs

What a combination this is. Sweet, tangy, salty – no taste bud will come away disappointed! And it's so easy to knock up as well, that's what we call a win-win around here.

makes 2

360kcal per serving

⅓ x 320g packet chilled ready-rolled puff pastry sheet (approx. 105g)

100g soft goats' cheese

3 tsp runny honey

2 ripe fresh figs, quartered

A little finely chopped rosemary

2 pinches of salt

1 Preheat the oven to 180°C/160°C fan/Gas Mark 4. Line a small baking tray with greaseproof paper.

2 Take the puff pastry and split it in half, so you get 2 rough squares of pastry. Carefully score a line about 1cm in all the way around each piece, but don't cut all the way through. Fold the edges over so you create a little puff pastry border around each piece. Place them on the lined baking tray, then pop in the oven for around 8 minutes, until lightly golden and puffed up.

3 While they cook, add the goats' cheese and 2 teaspoons of the honey into a bowl and give it a good beating to combine.

4 Remove the pastry from the oven, press the puffed-up centre parts of each square down, leaving the border raised. Share the goats' cheese mix between each pastry case and spread it out, topping each with the fig quarters, a pinch or two of chopped rosemary and a pinch of salt.

5 Return to the oven for another 7–8 minutes, until the sides are golden brown and crisp.

6 Remove from the oven and drizzle the remaining 1 teaspoon of honey across the puffs before tucking in.

no-faff falafel bites

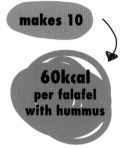

makes 10

60kcal per falafel with hummus

These really can be called no-faff, as they can be in the oven and cooking away in 5 minutes. And the hummus is just as easy as well and packs a lovely pepper punch. Serve the falafels up with a bowl of the hummus and let all your friends dig in.

For the falafels

1 x 400g tin chickpeas, drained and rinsed

A large handful of parsley, chopped

1 garlic clove, roughly chopped

1 tsp ground cumin

1 tsp ground coriander

1 tbsp plain flour

1 tsp olive oil

Salt and ground black pepper

For the hummus

80g (drained weight) tinned chickpeas, drained and rinsed

20g (drained weight) roasted red pepper from a jar, drained and chopped

1 tsp tahini

A squeeze of lemon juice

1 tsp extra virgin olive oil

1 Preheat the oven to 150°C/130°C fan/Gas Mark 2. Line a baking tray with greaseproof paper.

2 Add all the falafel ingredients, except the oil, into a food processor along with a good pinch of salt and pepper and get that whizzing away. The mix will get very crumbly as everything combines, so stop every now and then to scrape down the sides. When you can take a tablespoon-size amount and roll it into a ball and it holds together well, you are ready. Add a splash of water to the mix if required.

3 Carefully make roughly ping pong ball-sized balls from the mix and place them on to the lined baking tray, you should get 10 good-sized falafels. Drizzle or spray them with the oil and then pop in the oven for 20 minutes, or until lovely and golden.

4 While they cook, clean out the food processor and then add all the hummus ingredients, except the oil, along with a pinch of salt and pepper. Start the processor off and, once everything is well combined, drizzle in the oil until you get a lovely creamy hummus. Transfer to a serving dish.

5 When the falafels are ready, serve and use them to scoop up that lovely hummus.

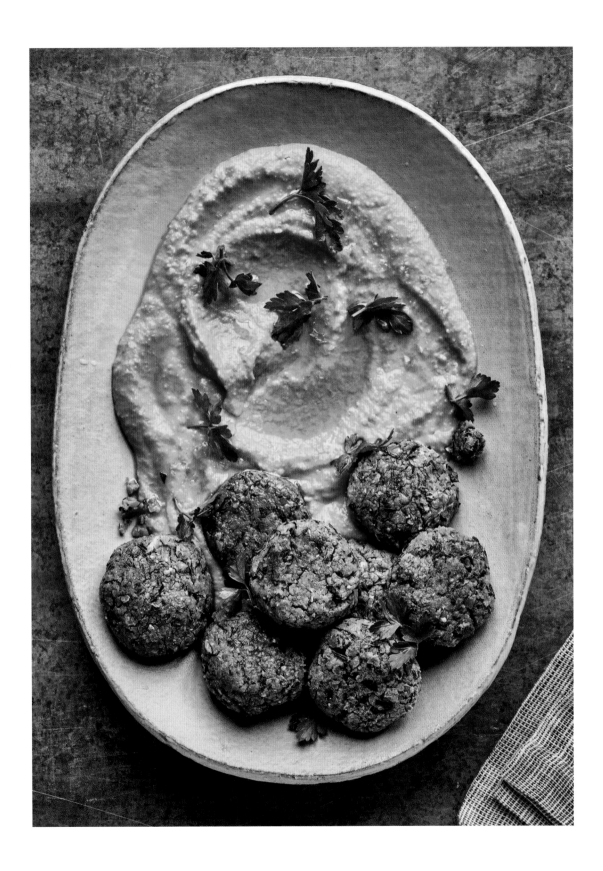

rocking croquettes

These are crispy little snacks of joy! Packed full of fresh flavours, and perfect to pass around at a party. Even better, they look like they were tricky to knock up so will impress all your friends, but really they couldn't be easier!

350g sweet potatoes

2 spring onions, finely chopped

A large handful of coriander, finely chopped

Grated zest of ½ lemon

1 tbsp hot sauce (optional)

1 x 110g tin of drained tuna

1 tbsp plain flour

1 medium egg

40g panko breadcrumbs

1 tsp olive oil

Salt and ground black pepper

Sweet chilli sauce (page 235), to serve

1 Pop the sweet potatoes on to a microwaveable plate or bowl and whack in the microwave on High for 4 minutes. Carefully give them a squeeze (they will be hot!) to see if they are nice and soft, if not, give them another minute or so and test again (thicker potatoes may need microwaving for up to 8–10 minutes in total). When they're lovely and soft, remove and leave to cool a little.

2 When cool enough to handle, peel away the skins and discard, then add the potato flesh to a bowl along with the spring onions, coriander, lemon zest, hot sauce and tuna. Give that a really good mix so it is combined, then divide into 9 equal portions and carefully roll each one into a chunky cigar-shaped croquette. Pop them on a plate and into the fridge for 10 minutes to set.

3 Preheat the oven to 170°C/150°C fan/Gas Mark 3½. Line a baking tray with greaseproof paper.

4 Add the flour to a plate, season with salt and pepper and give that a little mix together. Crack the egg into a large bowl and whisk, and place the breadcrumbs on to another plate.

5 Now it's just a case of dipping the croquettes, one at a time, in the flour (shaking off any excess), then into the egg and finally into the breadcrumbs to coat. Pop each one on to the lined baking tray.

6 When all the croquettes are breaded, spray or drizzle with the oil and bake for 15–20 minutes, until golden. Serve them up with the sweet chilli sauce.

spring rolls

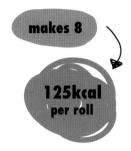

Not your greasy, bland spring rolls either! Full of fresh veggies, packed with flavour from soy and teriyaki sauces, and then baked instead of fried to keep them light and delicious. And much lower on the calorie front, too.

1 tbsp vegetable oil,
plus extra for brushing

3 garlic cloves,
finely diced

1 tbsp peeled and finely
diced fresh root ginger

150g Savoy cabbage,
chopped

150g mushrooms,
chopped

100g baby corn,
chopped

100g carrots, chopped

70g bean sprouts

2 tbsp light soy sauce

2 tbsp teriyaki sauce

8 spring roll wrappers
(not rice paper
wrappers)

3 tbsp sweet chilli
sauce (page 235)

1 Add the oil to a wok over a high heat, then add in the garlic, ginger and all the vegetables and stir-fry for a few minutes to start to soften the veg. Add the soy and teriyaki sauces and continue to stir-fry until the sauce is absorbed and the mix is thick, about 4–5 minutes. Remove from the wok to a plate and leave to cool completely.

2 Preheat the oven to 170°C/150°C fan/Gas Mark 3½. Lightly oil a baking tray.

3 Once the veg mix is cool, fill your spring roll wrappers. To do this, lay the wrappers out, one at a time (keeping the rest covered so they don't dry out), on a board or work surface, share the veg mix between the wrappers, then roll each one up to enclose the filling, tucking the ends in as you go.

4 Place the spring rolls on the oiled baking tray, brush with a little more oil, then bake for 15–20 minutes, until golden and crisp.

5 Serve the spring rolls hot from the oven with the sweet chilli sauce on the side.

courgette and feta blinis with herby yogurt

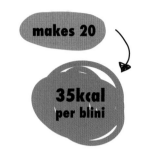

makes 20

35kcal
per blini

*These little discs of joy are the ultimate party snack.
Light and fluffy blinis, packed with lovely herby
flavours, and a delicious dip to go alongside them.
It's worth having a party just to make a batch of them!*

For the blinis
250g courgettes, grated
50g feta cheese,
  crumbled
½ tbsp chopped dill
A few mint leaves,
  chopped
2 tbsp plain flour
1 tsp baking powder
2 medium eggs
1 tbsp vegetable oil
Salt and ground
  black pepper

For the herby yogurt
100g natural yogurt
½ tbsp chopped dill
A few mint leaves,
  chopped

1 Make the blinis. Place the grated courgette into a clean tea towel, then squeeze out as much of the water from it as you can. Pop the courgette back into a large bowl.

2 Add in the well-crumbled feta along with the dill, mint, flour and baking powder as well as a good pinch of salt and pepper. Give that all a good mix, then whisk the eggs in a separate bowl before pouring in. Stir well to combine; you will end up with a chunky batter.

3 Place a large frying pan over a medium heat and add the oil. When hot, spoon in teaspoon-size amounts of the batter, pressing down to form rough circles approximately 2cm across (you may need to do this in a couple of batches, depending on the size of your pan). Let them cook away for around 3–4 minutes on each side, or until golden brown.

4 Meanwhile, stir the yogurt and herbs together in a small bowl.

5 Pile all the blinis on to a serving plate and serve up with the herby yogurt alongside.

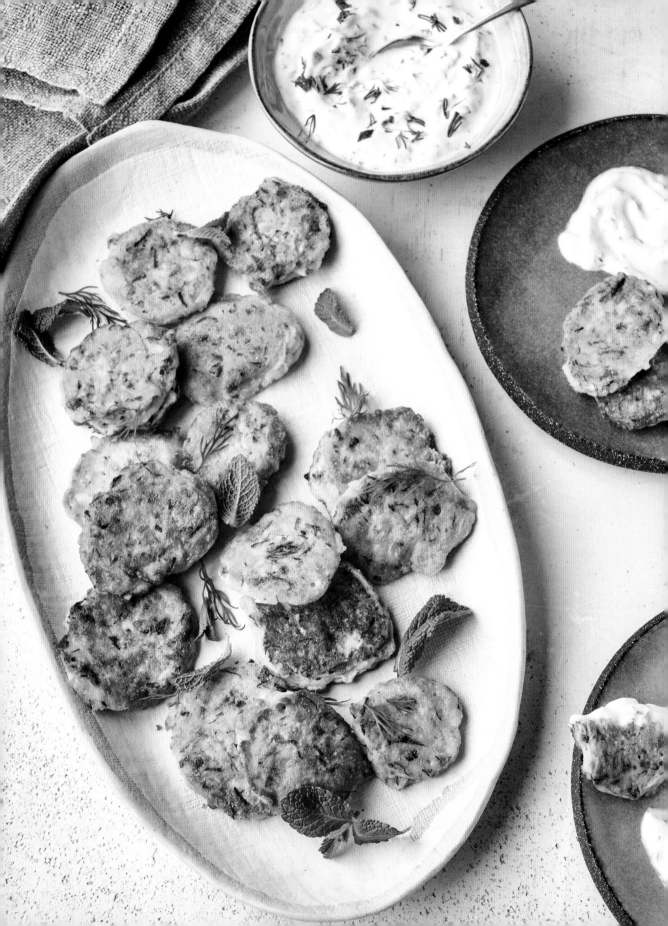

stunning sides

kimchi

makes 500g

One of the world's best condiments here! Just a spoonful can transform a meal from average to exceptional, and don't think it's just for Korean food either. Topping a burger, packed into a cheese sarnie, even stuffed in a tortilla, you will be finding ways to add it to almost everything!

For the kimchi base

1 white onion, quartered

2 large garlic cloves, peeled

1 thumb-sized piece of fresh root ginger, peeled

2 tsp chilli powder (or to taste)

For classic kimchi (130kcal for the whole lot)

500g Chinese leaf cabbage, roughly chopped

10g sea salt

For spinach, carrot and apple kimchi (230kcal for the whole lot)

200g fresh spinach

200g carrots, grated

100g dessert apples, cored and grated

10g sea salt

1 Start by making the kimchi base by adding all the ingredients to a food processor and whizzing until everything is finely chopped. Add a splash of water to help it to break down.

2 You now need to prepare the cabbage or veg/fruit elements. Add the chosen ingredients to a large bowl along with the salt and give it a really good massage so the salt gets combined. Squeeze and scrunch it all together and don't be shy, you want to work it all quite hard. Leave the veg for 10 minutes, during which time the water in the veg will start to come out.

3 Now it's just a case of adding in the kimchi base mix to the veg, then giving everything a really good mix and squeeze together again. There should be a fair bit of liquid when you squeeze the veg now, which is perfect.

4 Add the lot, veg, water, everything, into a clean and sterilised 500g glass jar (page 230). Pack it all in as you add it so there are no air pockets, then top up with just enough cold water so that everything is covered. Put the lid on the jar. You now just need to leave it for around a week at a cool room temperature for the fermentation to occur before serving. Once reopened, the kimchi will keep for at least 2 weeks in the fridge.

pickled courgettes

These are a bit of a secret obsession of ours! They are so unbelievably easy to make, but they taste so good. And you'll soon be finding any excuse to add them into your meals. We have given you an idea for how to use them on page 126, but that's just the tip of the iceberg!

2 courgettes, thinly
sliced (approximately
250g total weight)

½ red onion, thinly sliced

1 red chilli, deseeded
and thinly sliced

250ml white wine vinegar

1 Preheat the oven to 150°C/130°C fan/Gas Mark 2.

2 Sterilise a clean, large glass jar by washing and rinsing it, then placing it in the oven for about 10 minutes. Remove and leave to cool slightly until you can handle it.

3 Now this couldn't be any easier. Just mix up the courgette, onion and chilli slices in a bowl, then pack them into the sterilised jar.

4 Combine the vinegar and 200ml of water in a jug, then pour into the jar so that all the veggies are covered. Seal the jar with a lid, then leave at a cool room temperature for at least 3 days but, ideally, for a week before you start tucking into them. Once opened, store in the fridge and use within 1 week.

mayonnaise

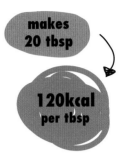

makes
20 tbsp

120kcal
per tbsp

The ultimate condiment — and when you make it yourself, it tastes so much better than a shop-bought version. But use it in moderation, it packs in the calories!

2 large egg yolks
½ tbsp Dijon mustard
240ml vegetable oil
1 tbsp white wine vinegar
2-4 tbsp hot sauce (or
  to taste) (optional)
Salt and ground
  black pepper

1 This recipe ideally needs to be made in a small food processor or with a stick blender. If you only have a large food processor, you will be better off whisking it by hand, and it will get your arms working!

2 Add the yolks into the food processor or into a large bowl along with the mustard and a pinch of salt and pepper. Give that a good whizz or a whisk for 30 seconds, then slowly start to drip in the oil. You want to do this as slowly as you can at the start, making sure the oil is being incorporated and you start to see the mixture fluff up and thicken, then you can start to drizzle it in a little quicker.

3 When you have incorporated all the oil, add the vinegar and continue to mix for a further 30 seconds, until you get a lovely light but thick texture.

4 For those of you who like it spicy, add the hot sauce now and fold that through the mayonnaise. Use as required.

5 This mayo will keep in a sterilised (page 230) and sealed jar in the fridge for up to a week.

red onion and chilli jam

This recipe is so easy but it delivers a real flavour punch. You'll see it used in the book but use your imagination with it, too! If you are thinking about using a shop-bought chutney or pickle, stick this in there instead!

1 tbsp olive oil
2 red onions, finely diced
½ red chilli, deseeded and finely diced
1 garlic clove, minced
1 tbsp light soft brown sugar
3 tbsp balsamic vinegar
Salt and ground black pepper

1 Place a small saucepan over a medium-low heat and add the oil, then the onions and chilli. Let that cook very gently for around 10–15 minutes, stirring regularly to ensure the mix doesn't catch.

2 Next, add in the garlic and sugar along with a good pinch of salt and pepper. Give that a stir to combine and continue to cook gently for another 2–3 minutes before adding the vinegar. Turn the heat up a little and let that bubble away until the vinegar has evaporated and the jam is lovely and thick.

3 Remove from the heat and allow to cool slightly before transferring to a sterilised 125g jam jar (page 230). Seal the jar with a lid and store in the fridge.

4 This will keep well in the fridge for at least a month, so make as big a batch as you like by just multiplying the ingredients by the number of portions required.

burger sauce

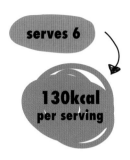

serves 6

130kcal
per serving

We were pretty pleased with John when he perfected this one! Those golden arches do have a great sauce, but this is about as good a homemade version as we have tasted. It's also amazingly simple, so that's even better.

100g mayonnaise
  (page 231)
10g American mustard
½ tsp cider vinegar
¼ tsp garlic powder
¼ tsp onion powder
½ tsp smoked paprika
1 gherkin, drained
  and finely diced

1 Grab yourself a bowl and add all the ingredients, then give that a good mix up to make sure everything gets combined. That's it! So simple but so good.

2 This sauce will keep in a sterilised (page 230) and sealed jar in the fridge for up to 1 week.

Top Tip: Want to make this vegan? Just use a shop-bought vegan mayonnaise in place of ours, which will change the calories to 110kcal per serving.

mango chutney

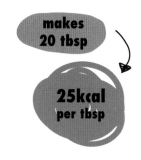

makes
20 tbsp

25kcal
per tbsp

OK, so you can basically get this anywhere and use it straight from the jar. But there is something a little bit special about making your own, and it also allows you to be creative, using the perfect blend of spices for your own taste buds.

½ tsp vegetable oil

1 small garlic
  clove, minced

½ tsp peeled and minced
  fresh root ginger

½ small red chilli,
  deseeded and
  finely chopped

½ tsp nigella seeds

¼ tsp ground coriander

A pinch of ground
  turmeric

A pinch of ground cumin

A pinch of ground
  cinnamon

A pinch of salt

250g frozen mango
  chunks

60ml white wine vinegar

60g granulated sugar

1 Add the oil to a saucepan and place over a medium-low heat. When hot, add in the garlic, ginger and chilli and fry for 2 minutes. Add in all the spices and the salt and give it all a good stir to combine. Let that fry away for a further 1–2 minutes.

2 Now it's just a case of adding the rest of the ingredients, then stir well to combine and bring that to the boil. Drop the heat to low and simmer, uncovered, for around 30 minutes or until lovely and thick, breaking up any larger chunks of mango as it cooks.

3 Once it's ready, transfer the chutney to a sterilised 300ml jar (page 230) and seal with a lid. Leave to cool, then store in the fridge. This will keep in the fridge for up to a month.

sweet chilli sauce

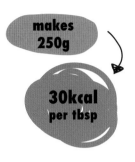

makes 250g

30kcal per tbsp

The ultimate flavour boosting condiment! It's not just for Asian inspired dishes though. Pop it on a toasted cheese sandwich or drizzle over some cooked bacon, use your imagination and find your own favourites!

110g granulated sugar

60ml white wine vinegar

1 large garlic clove, finely diced

60g red chillies, diced (see Top Tip)

½ tbsp cornflour

1 Add the sugar, vinegar, garlic and chillies along with 125ml of water to a saucepan and place over a medium heat. Bring to the boil, then leave it to simmer, uncovered, for 10 minutes.

2 In a separate bowl, mix the cornflour with 1 tablespoon of water, then add this to the sauce and simmer for a further 3 minutes, stirring, until the sauce thickens.

3 Leave to cool for a few minutes, then transfer to a sterilised jam jar (page 230) and seal with a lid. Leave to cool, then store in a cool, dry place for up to 6 months.

4 Once opened, store in the fridge and use within 1 month.

Top Tip: For a slightly less spicy version, remove the seeds from the chillies before dicing.

index

acknowledgements

The whole team at #itsfine would like to thank Clare and our publishers, Orion, for believing in our movement and identifying with how important it was to write this book to shake up the dieting industry once and for all.

I would like to dedicate this book to my wife, Cara, for her unconditional belief, support and love, and for giving me the confidence to create something I was so scared of doing for years. Alfie, you motivate me every day to make a difference in the world and work as hard as I can. Mum, stay strong, stay positive, you've got this. **Ben**

Firstly, I want to share my gratitude to Ben and his unrivalled passion for this industry and for wanting to join forces with me to help people discover food freedom! Our paths crossed at the perfect time and creating #itsfine has been such an amazing journey. A big thank you to my manager, Claire, for making this happen, as always, I'm so grateful for your support and friendship. Lastly, I want to dedicate this book to all of you who have struggled as a result of following a fad diet – you deserve so much more, and I truly hope this book will help you. **Pete**

credits

Recipes: John Burrows
Publisher: Vicky Eribo
Editor: George Brooker
Project Editor: Susie Bertinshaw
Photography: Chris Terry
Food Styling: Lou Kenney
Prop Styling: Faye Wears
Design and Art Direction: Helen Ewing;
   Abi Hartshorne (hartstudio.co.uk)
Copy-editor: Anne Sheasby
Proofreader: Jane Howard
Indexer: Ingrid Lock
Production Controller: Sarah Cook